SWARNA MOLDANADO, PhD, MPH
ALEX MOLDANADO, MD

KILLER DISEASES, MODERN-DAY EPIDEMICS

Keys to Stopping
Heart Disease, Diabetes,
Cancer, and Obesity
in Their Tracks

Basic
Health
PUBLICATIONS, INC.

Basic Health Publications, Inc.
an imprint of Turner Publishing Company
Nashville, TN
www.turnerpublishing.com

Library of Congress Cataloging-in-Publication Data is available through the Library of Congress.

Interior design: Gary A. Rosenberg
Cover design: Maddie Cothren
Cover image: Lightspring/Shutterstock.com

Printed in the United States of America

10   9   8   7   6   5   4   3   2   1

Contents

PART 3
Keeping Chronic Diseases at Bay
or Stopping Them in Their Tracks

For Our Parents

and

Our Son Arjun

*With Gratitude for His Service
to Our Country*

Acknowledgments

We would like to acknowledge the superb editing of much of this book by Roberta Waddell, and express our gratitude to her. We would like to give our thanks to the phenomenal jobs done by Maddie Cothren and Gary Rosenberg for the book cover and interior design respectively and Jon O'Neal, the managing editor at Turner Publishing, for making certain that the book is the best it can be for the reader. We would also like to express our gratitude to Dr. Lawrence Lenhart, for reviewing the chapter on cardiovascular diseases and offering many thoughtful comments and suggestions that added to the chapter. Dr. Lenhart is an experienced physician, who practiced internal medicine and cardiology in San Mateo, California. We would like to express our thanks to our friend Vijay Narula, an experienced nurse and a certified diabetes educator, for her review of the content on diabetes, and offering helpful suggestions. We would be remiss if we did not acknowledge the support and encouragement we received from many friends and family for the first author's earlier book on legumes that spurred us to write this book.

Swarna Moldanado
Alex Moldanado

Preface

Today, thanks to both an ever-increasing body of knowledge about diseases, and more and better ways of disseminating this information, we know more about the causes, best treatment practices, and management of many of the diseases that beset us than at any other time in history. The information is generated worldwide through research in medicine, and the basic sciences. Much of the research that contributes to this growing body of knowledge is paid for by public monies to facilitate scientific inquiry into the causes and new treatment modalities for diseases that take a toll on public health. Yet the information generated mostly remains enshrined in medical and other professional journals, which are often written in technical language, and are laden with medical and scientific jargon, and complex statistical analyses and terms meant strictly for the consumption of medical, and other highly trained professionals. The public is often left to glean what they can from the print and sound bites of mass media that generally cover only the newsworthy and trendy health topics. People are also increasingly flocking to the Internet for health information that can be conflicting, confusing, and even bewildering to those not in the healthcare field. The resulting ambiguity can have the unintended effect of causing the public to lose faith in the message the information is intended to deliver. People are entitled to credible, usable, health-related information that is conveyed in clear, non-technical language so a layperson can easily grasp and receive the health message. While there are an increasing number of publications on the market, popular magazines among them, that address health topics catering to the lay public, the topic of disease prevention is not a common thread among them. Promoting an understanding of how and why chronic diseases set in and progress, we believe, not only demystifies that process, but is also likely to spur actions that promote health and prevent illness.

As two-health professionals—one with a background in nursing and public health, and the other in medicine, we have long subscribed to the notion that health education is one of the most valuable tools that health professionals have at their disposal to use for the benefit of their patients and the community at large. Yet it seldom is used to its full potential to achieve health promotion and disease prevention at the individual or at the aggregate level. While the Affordable Care Act enacted in the U.S. in recent years is intended to improve access to affordable and accessible quality healthcare, including preventive care, it can only fully succeed in its mission if an informed public avails itself of the preventive healthcare services, and simultaneously adopts health-promoting and disease-preventing health behaviors. A basic requirement of this alternate orientation to health behavior is an unambiguous message that most diseases are preventable at various stages in their progression, *including before they ever set in.* This book is specifically intended to help the reader understand the concepts related to the development and progression of chronic diseases, and become aware of the opportunities for detecting and ultimately preventing these diseases.

The book contains 10 chapters, plus an introduction and summary. The first three chapters address concepts related to disease development, such as the key players that cause disease, the exposure to risk factors for disease, and preventing or intercepting disease through avoiding and/or minimizing exposure to risk. The incidence, prevalence and causes of the major chronic diseases that account for the most deaths and healthcare costs—cardiovascular diseases, cancers, diabetes, and obesity, are covered in the next four chapters. Each one of these chapters includes one or more case histories, contributed by the physician co-author, Dr. Alex Moldanado, who is a practicing family physician. The cases are all patients from his practice, with the names altered to protect their privacy, and are intended to illustrate the concepts described in the book. Lifestyle choices that have a proven connection with health and disease, and thus warrant making and keeping them for life are detailed in chapter eight. Chapter nine describes the preventive health services, including specific screening tests appropriate for different age, sex, and risk profiles that play a key role in intercepting the chronic diseases through early detection and intervention. The last chapter describes the disease burden of chronic diseases addressed in the book, from an individual, family, and societal perspective. The summary ties the salient points of the content covered, and highlights the message of the book—killer chronic diseases can be prevented before they ever set in, or stopped in their tracks by adopting, and adhering to, the right lifestyle choices.

Swarna Moldanado, Ph.D., M.P.H.
Alex Moldanado, M.D.

Introduction

The United States is among the wealthiest nations in the world and spends more as a percentage of its gross domestic product (GDP) on healthcare than any other country in the developed world, but it is not the healthiest country in the world. Although life expectancy and survival rates in the United States have improved dramatically over the past century, Americans experience higher rates of disease and injury and die earlier than people in other developed countries, according to a report released in 2013 by the National Research Council and the Institute of Medicine.[1] The report points to an alarming fact that more people in the U.S. die before their fiftieth birthday than in any other developed country, and that the mortality gap between the U.S. and other rich countries is widening. Recent studies suggest that the U.S. health disadvantage persists across the person's lifespan, and across the socio-economic spectrum. Although this health disadvantage has been increasing for decades, the scale of this disparity in the U.S., relative to its peer countries, is becoming more apparent as death and illness rates from chronic diseases like heart disease, cancer, type-2 diabetes, and obesity have reached epidemic proportions, and are taking a heavy toll on public health in the U.S.

Health and illness are two dynamic states on a continuum that behave like a see-saw, as one goes up the other goes down. In other words, you can't be both healthy and ill at the same time. In most instances, it is possible to transition back and forth between the two states. When you come down with a self-resolving illness like the common cold, you return to the state of being healthy again rather quickly. But that is not the case with chronic diseases, such as heart disease, cancer, diabetes, or a major injury that results in significant pathological changes in the body and requires intervention, often over an extended period of time, and in some cases for the remainder of the person's life. The duration and severity of illness depend on how quickly the disease is detected and intervened. For some, the damage already caused by the disease may be irreversible, but advances in medical therapy and technology make it possible to live a fairly normal and productive life even with the residual damage. Most diseases (unlike injuries) are rarely sudden events, providing opportunities at various stages in their development to intercept and/or arrest the progress, including before they ever set in. A fundamental understanding of the factors that come together to predispose a person to a disease can aid in taking steps to prevent it, or at least intercept it as early in its progression as possible, so the ill effects of the disease are minimized.

It is commonly known that when a disease is detected early, the prognosis is generally better than when it is detected late and has progressed to a more advanced stage. Perhaps a less well-known fact is that many diseases lend themselves to being intercepted at various stages in their progression, including before they ever start. Epidemiologists, the public health professionals who study the distribution and determinants of health and disease, have long known that diseases, both infectious and non-infectious, follow a course that is normal for them. They called it the *natural history* of a disease—a term that describes identifiable stages spanning the progression of a particular disease. Everyone has probably heard someone say that a relative or someone they knew had suddenly died of a massive heart attack while just sitting and reading a newspaper, or somebody who they thought was a picture of good health had just been diagnosed with stage IV cancer. Epidemiologists argue that the seeming suddenness of these events is not sudden at all, and that each is merely the culmination of a process that had been in the making, quite possibly for a long time. In some diseases, for example heart disease, the foundation is laid even in the person's childhood and continues to build, usually due to poor health habits that pose a risk for that or other diseases in later life. Autopsy studies done on U.S. servicemen killed in the Korean and Vietnam wars, as well as in the more recent wars in Iraq and Afghanistan, have provided evidence that coronary heart disease begins at a young age.[2] In these young (average age 25.9 years), otherwise healthy, individuals, atherosclerosis (hardening of the arteries) was found in the coronary artery that supplies blood to the heart, and the severity varied by age and the number and kind of cardiovascular risk factors the person was exposed to. In general, the older the individual, and the more risk factors, such as previously detected abnormal levels of cholesterol, uncontrolled hypertension (abnormally and chronically elevated blood pressure), and the amount of overweight, the greater was the severity of atherosclerosis. Hardening of the arteries has also been reported from autopsies done on young civilian individuals who died from accidental injuries or were homicide victims. This knowledge not only points to the need for targeting chronic disease prevention to a young population, but also to the fact that early prevention holds the most promise in averting the disease in the future.

Up until about the mid-twentieth century, infectious diseases, such as typhoid, cholera, polio, tuberculosis, and respiratory and gastrointestinal infections, caused the most deaths, resulting in an average life expectancy as low as forty-seven years at the turn of the century. Those diseases were conquered in the second half of the twentieth century through relatively simple means—improvements in environmental sanitation, safe drinking water and food, immunizations, and the use of antibiotics like penicillin. These achievements, coupled with industrialization that led to an increased food supply, advances in technology, and more and better medicines, caused life expectancy to rise at an accelerated pace. However, as people started to live longer, a new crop of non-infectious diseases came in to replace the infectious diseases as major killers. They are called *degenerative diseases* because of the progressive tissue-damaging effect they have on the body. Prime examples include the *cardiovascular diseases* that kill more men and women than any other disease group and are responsible for one in four of all deaths in the U.S. *Cancer* (all types) causes the second highest number of deaths. Deaths from *strokes* and *type-2 diabetes* rank as the fourth and seventh among the top ten causes of death in the U.S.[3] Today, cardiovascular diseases, cancer, and type-2 diabetes combined account for two of every three deaths in the United States. In contrast, as noted, in the early part of the twentieth century the three leading causes of death in the United States were all infectious diseases—pneumonia, tuberculosis, and diarrhea. Since the average life expectancy was very low at the time, many people did not live long enough to develop the chronic diseases—heart disease, cancer, or adult-onset diabetes—that account for the most deaths today. While the average life expectancy in the United States rose steadily in the latter half of the twentieth century, and people are living longer, they are not necessarily living free of disease in their middle and later years. The diseases many now experience during their middle and later years are chronic, often debilitating in nature, robbing them of their health and vitality, disrupting their lives and often that of their loved ones, and posing an economic burden on the family and society. The knowledge gained to date about the causes of these disease conditions and the associated risk factors offers opportunity and promise for prevention, as well as early detection, so the damage, both potential and real, can be minimized. Yet, attention to disease prevention is falling far short of its potential, both at the individual and aggregate levels. Despite the strong, incontrovertible evidence supporting investment of resources in disease prevention, it is estimated that less than 3 cents out of every healthcare dollar is spent on prevention in the U.S. The low investment in disease prevention and health promotion also promotes, and cements, the belief among the public that diseases cannot truly be prevented, and if you are unlucky enough to develop one, you go seek treatment and all will be well and good. Despite being called *healthcare,* the model being used and championed by the healthcare delivery system is one of *sick care.* This model of care also squarely places the control of an individual's health on external sources like doctors and hospitals, and not with the individual. This perhaps is the reason why so many people still smoke tobacco, fail to engage in any regular physical activity, eat poorly, and gain weight, despite knowing (or hearing) that these behaviors are detrimental to their health. A culture that embraces immediate gratification and shuns delayed gratification also poses a challenge for disease prevention, particularly at the individual level because the rewards of disease prevention are in the form of averted disease in the future, the often-distant future, and are invisible and not easy to fathom in the present, even by the most astute.

Most of us are familiar with the saying, "an ounce of prevention is worth a pound of cure." Although Benjamin Franklin originally coined the phrase in 1736 as fire-fighting advice, it is equally applicable, and possibly more so, in the case of disease prevention. While the property destroyed in fire (but not the lives lost) can be rebuilt, many preventable diseases, besides often requiring prolonged and costly treatments, can result in irreversible damage, a diminished quality of life, and even death in some cases. In the context of disease prevention, it is perhaps appropriate to amend the phrase to say, "a few ounces of prevention are worth life itself." Thanks to ever-advancing technology, with the information explosion as one of its many benefits, the average lay (non-medical) individual now has access to health information that was not possible just a few decades ago. Of course, having the right knowledge is not a guarantee it will be put to use when it comes to adopting habits conducive to promoting health and preventing disease. As implied in the book's title, a majority of diseases can be either prevented from ever taking root or intercepted at various points in their progression. In some instances, the damage already caused to the body by unhealthful practices may even be reversed—a prime example of such a reversal would come from giving up smoking. The relationship between sustained health habits and subsequent disease or death has been extensively studied, and research points to incontrovertible evidence of a strong relationship between the two.

In his book on longevity, *The Blue Zones: 9 Lessons for Living Longer from the People Who've Lived the Longest,* Dan Buettner, *The New York Times* best-selling author, describes the demonstrable evidence of such a relationship.[4] Buettner and his team identified five places in the world—Sardinia, Italy; Okinawa, Japan; Loma Linda, United States; Ikaria, Greece; and Nicoya, Costa Rica, where there are higher percentages of people not only living the longest, but also enjoying full and active lives well into their 90s and sometimes beyond. Buettner called these places the *Blue Zones*.

Lester Breslow and James Enstrom explored the relationship between seven personal health practices and the death rates among nearly 7,000 adults in Alameda County, California, over a period of 9.5 years.[5] The seven health practices they examined were: eating breakfast regularly, getting seven to eight hours of sleep a day, engaging in regular physical activity, never smoking cigarettes, moderate or no use of alcohol, maintaining proper weight, and not eating between meals. The two researchers found that the number of health practices observed by the participants in the study showed a strong inverse relationship with mortality, for men in particular. Men who followed all the seven health practices had a death rate that was 72 percent lower than men who engaged in health practices between zero and three. The women who followed all the seven health practices had a 57 percent reduction in their death rate, compared to women who followed three or fewer of the practices. The benefits from adherence to even some of the seven health practices attest to the power of the association between health habits and subsequent health and illness. It can also be deduced that the converse is true, and a failure to make and adhere to healthy lifestyle choices portends poor health. An exploration of how the cultivation and consistent practice of the right health habits can help promote health, and prevent or reduce the risk for major chronic diseases is the central theme of this book.

PART 1

Evolution of
a Chronic Disease

Part 1 introduces you to several key concepts in the development and progression of chronic disease. These include the multiple causation theory that focuses on the individual, the environment, and the interplay between the two; the natural history of a disease, the characteristic natural progression of a chronic disease; the modifiable and non-modifiable risk factors for disease, those you can avoid and the ones you have little or no control over; and lastly the connection between lifestyle and disease.

1

Disease in the Making

Since the mid-twentieth century, when global public health efforts resulted in greatly reducing, or in some cases eradicating, the incidence of killer communicable diseases, attention has been diverted to unraveling the causes of non-communicable diseases. This has resulted in the knowledge that disease is often the result of multiple factors interacting with one another, and seldom of a single factor operating alone. This new awareness explains why, when a room full of people is exposed to a person with a common cold, not everyone in the room will come down with a cold, but one or more people are likely to be infected. In this example, to become ill with a cold, you need a *host*-person without the cold, an *agent*—the cold virus (harbored by the person already infected), and an *environment*—the room where the host was exposed to the infected person. But even though all three factors were present for everyone in that room, not everyone will come down with a cold. The explanation for this quandary lies in the fact that the agent and the environmental factors are necessary, but not sufficient to cause disease. Furthermore, there are other factors embedded in each of the three key players that are constantly interacting with one another and ultimately creating conditions that are either optimal for resisting the disease or succumbing to it by the host. For over a century, this knowledge has aided preventive medicine and public health efforts in preventing many fatal and disabling diseases, such as polio, and has aided in the early detection and timely treatment of numerous others.

A key role in the development of this body of knowledge is played by epidemiologists, the public health professionals whose original job was to investigate communicable disease epidemics, assist in their prevention, and help control their spread in population groups. Once the major communicable diseases were conquered, or at least were on the wane, these public health professionals extended their investigations to trends and patterns in non-infectious diseases that were gradually taking the place of communicable diseases as major causes of illness and death. Examining the associations between broad arrays of factors believed to play a role in causing these diseases was central to this quest—some of their earliest research findings uncovered the association between health behavior and disease and death rates. The association they uncovered between cigarette smoking and lung cancer was a crowning achievement of these scientists. It eventually led to a campaign against cigarette advertisements, the sale of cigarettes to minors, and smoking in many public spaces, that began in the last decades of the twentieth century and continues to this day. This multi-faceted attempt to reduce smoking rates was achieved despite the major tobacco companies with deep pockets countering their efforts by challenging the scientific conclusion that cigarette smoking caused lung cancer. They did so by exploiting the fact that the ethics of research would preclude a randomized control trial, a gold standard in clinical research that would have entailed randomly assigning a group of non-smokers to smoke in order to establish a cause-and-effect relationship between smoking and lung cancer. The resistance from tobacco companies worked in their favor for a while until the opposing evidence put forth by the scientific community overwhelmed the corporate rationale.

The early disease-causation model was centered on infectious diseases, consisting of the host-human or animal affected by the disease, the agent, mainly disease-causing microbes, and the environment that both the host and the agent inhabited. The study of non-infectious diseases in later years led epidemiologists to theorize that although the three elements were necessary, they were not sufficient to cause disease, a phrase they are fond of using. The reason for this evolution in thinking was a growing evidence that all diseases cannot be attributed to a single cause or factor, but are the result of multiple factors that interact with one another, and not necessarily in the same manner in every individual affected by a disease condition. Thus was born the *theory of multiple causation* in the onset of disease that has become central to the contemporary public-health efforts to combat disease. This concept redirects the focus from a single factor like a disease-causing microorganism, to a combination of interacting factors within the individual and the environment, whose combined effect may be greater than that caused by the sum of individual ones, due to their synergistic nature.

KEY PLAYERS IN DISEASE CAUSATION

The Person

There are certain characteristics that individuals are born with, such as gender, race, and ethnicity, which carry with them a predisposition for certain specific diseases. Examples include women being uniquely at risk for diseases associated with pregnancy and childbearing, African-Americans being at greater risk for sickle cell anemia, and Jews of Eastern European ancestry being at higher risk for Tay-Sachs disease. Race, and ethnicity-related diseases indicate a genetic component unique to those groups. Socio-economic status, a composite index of years of schooling, occupation, and income, is increasingly recognized as playing a significant role in determining a person's health status. It exerts an indirect influence on health through such factors as access to safe and adequate housing, access to healthcare, nutritious food, amenities for leisure-time activities, and quality education. The year of birth also plays a role in determining how long, on average, a person from that cohort is expected to live, what diseases the person may be exposed to, what immunizations that confer immunity against certain diseases the person may receive, and finally what technological advances in diagnoses and treatments the individual may benefit from. The influence of age on both disease and death rates is seen in every age bracket beginning at birth. The first twenty-eight days after birth, referred to in the medical field as the *neonatal* period, are a critical period associated with high risk for death. During this period, the causes of death among newborns are primarily associated with complications from the birth process, birth defects, as well as a lack of adequate prenatal care, resulting in failure to detect and treat poor health conditions in the mother and baby during the gestation period. Thanks to tremendous advances in medicine in general, and neonatal care in particular, the death rate in this age group has been steadily declining for the past several decades.

Among children, the next critical period for contracting disease is between the ages of five and nine when typical childhood diseases—chicken pox, measles, and mumps—can strike. It is worth remembering that not so long ago the dreaded diseases of polio, diphtheria, whooping cough, and tetanus were also among the so-called childhood diseases that children were susceptible to—poliomyelitis, for example, left many dead or partially paralyzed. It was only due to successful campaigns of prevention and immunizations against these devastating diseases that many children survived who would not otherwise have.

Herd immunity, a concept that describes the resistance of a group to invasion and person-to-person spread of an infectious agent, relies on the immunity of a high proportion of individual members of a group to an infectious disease. During the course of an epidemic, when more than the usual number of people is infected with communicable diseases, such as chickenpox or measles, a number of susceptible individuals come down with the disease and spread it to others. Since the diseased individuals do develop immunity, as the epidemic progresses, the proportion of those with immunity relative to those without increases and the chance for person-to-person spread of the infection declines. After doing comparative studies of groups with high and low rates of immunization, public health authorities have determined that *herd immunity* is protective when at least 80 percent of the individual members of a group are immune to a disease, either by having had the disease or through immunization, preferably the latter. As some parents are refusing to have their children immunized, falsely believing that the mercury used as preservative in vaccines is responsible for a rise in the incidence of autism, many healthcare practitioners believe the *herd immunity* may be threatened. Multiple rigorous scientific studies have failed to find any link between the preservative used in vaccines and autism to date.[1] The outbreak of measles among children in the U.S. in 2014 is a painful reminder of what is likely if the herd immunity is diminished in a population. The centers for Disease Control and Prevention (CDC) reported that nearly 90 percent of the children who contracted measles during that outbreak were those who were either not vaccinated or whose vaccination status was not known.

The next age group at risk, primarily for injury and death from accidents, vehicular accidents in particular, is between sixteen and twenty-five years of age. This is associated with risk-taking behaviors in this age group, such as driving at high speed, driving under the influence, not consistently wearing seat belts or helmets, and in recent years the use of cell phone to talk and text while driving. Societal measures, such as enforcement of seat belt and helmet laws, anti-drunk-driving laws, bans on hand-held cellphone use while driving, and lowered speed limits, go a long way in preventing or reducing serious injuries. Finally, death rates are highest among the advanced age groups, and can be attributed to such chronic diseases as cancer, heart disease, and stroke. Although gender, race, ethnicity, and age are not regarded as risk factors that can be modified, the diseases and injuries associated with them are not always inevitable. Many lend themselves to early detection of the disease itself or a predisposition to it with genetic testing, which can then help guide decisions about intervention with prophylactic measures.

There are also many risk factors within the control of the person that determine whether that person succumbs to a certain disease, is able to keep it at bay for a lifetime, or can delay it for an extended period of time. These are often referred to as *lifestyle* choices. They include such things as tobacco use, alcohol consumption, diet, physical activity, adequate rest and sleep, stress management, family and personal relationships, and the timely use of preventive health services. The amount and the length (in years) of smoking, for example, not only increase the risk for diseases like lung cancer, heart disease, and emphysema, but also increase the person's susceptibility to other illnesses. Both a high-fat diet and physical inactivity contribute to weight gain, which over time can put a person at increased risk for diseases, such as heart disease, adult-onset diabetes, high blood pressure, arthritis, and some types of cancers. A lack of adequate rest, persistent dissatisfaction with a job or personal relationships, or an inability to manage stress effectively can place a person at risk for chronic fatigue, depression, and other mental health problems. Certain types of behaviors have also long been associated with being at higher risk for some diseases. For example, type A personality, characterized by drive and aggressive tendencies, is implicated in heart disease, and certain gastrointestinal diseases such as ulcerative colitis and irritable bowel syndrome. The link is attributed to personality-driven health behaviors like ineffective coping, poor interpersonal relationships, and inadequate rest and relaxation that result in high stress.

The Environment

The environment of an individual encompasses physical, biological, chemical, psychological, socioeconomic, and cultural components that can confer health benefits or health hazards. The individual's physical environment consists of many things—housing, population density, climate that can include extreme heat or cold, terrain, access to safe food, water, and transportation, exposure to hazards like industrial waste, noise and air pollution, and natural disasters, as well as school or work environments that can pose occupational hazards. Many environmental factors have a direct impact on the health of individuals and communities living in certain geographic areas. Lead poisoning in children, for example, has been linked to deteriorating houses, especially those with peeling wall paint, built prior to 1978 when paints containing lead were used. Similarly, a rising incidence of asthma, particularly among children living in low-income areas, is linked to higher concentrations of circulating pollutants in the air.

Living in proximity to a nuclear power plant can be hazardous to health, as has been demonstrated in several incidences around the world in recent history. In 2011, the earthquake triggered by a tsunami caused the Fukushima Daiichi Nuclear Power Plant in Japan to release a large amount of radioactive material into the environment. The explosions at Chernobyl's nuclear reactor in 1986 in Ukraine caused several deaths and exposed an undetermined number of people to radiation, as did the partial nuclear meltdown at the Three Mile Island nuclear power plant in Pennsylvania in 1979. Although these three accidents did not result in massive casualties, and no cases of cancer could be attributed to radiation exposure from the plants, all three serve as reminders of the potential health hazard of living close to a nuclear power plant.

Injury and death from occupational hazards like working with farm equipment or machines in factories, firefighting, and other rescue operations are not uncommon. Occupational health and safety regulations and compliance monitoring are aimed at reducing their incidence. Disease- or injury-producing physical agents include extreme heat or cold, radiation, very high altitude, as well as natural disasters, such as tsunamis, earthquakes, floods, and fires. The exposure to, and impact from, a physical agent can be sudden, as is likely in natural disasters, or slow, as in gradual and prolonged exposure to radiation.

A biological environment includes all of the living creatures (plants and animals) that share the planet, some of whom pose a threat to human health, either directly or by being carriers of disease. In the era of a high incidences of major communicable diseases, the biological environment played a more prominent role because the disease-causing microbes were able to flourish due to the lack of beneficial environmental sanitation (safe waste disposal, safe drinking water), inadequate housing, and high population density in urban areas that promoted their spread from person to person. At the present time, this is less of a factor in developed countries like the United States, but poor environmental sanitation, and inadequate access to safe food and water continue to pose the threat of infectious diseases in many developing countries. In West Africa, the recent resurgence of the infectious disease caused by Ebola virus is one such example that has the potential to spread beyond that continent, unless it is effectively contained with proper public health measures. For now, Ebola seems to be ebbing, but so is research into ways of stopping it, so there's always the chance it could resurface as a major threat down the road. Another emerging threat is a rise in the number of disease-causing microorganisms that are developing resistance to the drugs used to combat them, requiring continual development of newer drugs just to keep pace with them.

Chemical disease-causing agents in the environment include drugs, both legal and illegal, poisons, pesticides, chemicals used in laboratories, factories, and agriculture, as well as chemicals used as weapons during war or other conflicts.

A psychological environment that can confer health benefits includes a safe, secure, and nurturing home, especially during the most formative years of life—infancy and early childhood—and age-appropriate stimulation to foster cognitive development and self-esteem. Conversely, a deprivation in any of these areas can lead to a range of emotional and psychological problems that can dog an individual, sometimes for a lifetime. Physical, emotional, or sexual abuse in childhood, or in later years, often leads to psychological and emotional problems, that can manifest in dysfunctional relationships, poor self-esteem, and sometimes psychosomatic illnesses.

The socioeconomic environment, although often thought of in economic terms, is more complex and is a composite of years of formal education, occupation, and income. In the United States, it does exert a powerful influence on health and illness as reflected in the differing levels of disease and death rates, as well as healthcare spending and the outcomes in different population groups. Overall, the rates of disease, disability, and death, are higher among the lower social classes than the higher social classes. The difference can largely be explained by such positive factors as access to safe and adequate housing, quality healthcare, healthier choices in food, abundant leisure-time activities, and such negative factors as exposure to environmental pollutants and violence. Much has been written about the connection between health and social class. Due to limited resources that have to be allocated to many competing needs, the poor are often oriented toward the present and the immediate. For anyone concerned about having enough money to pay the rent at the end of the month, even paying for health insurance may seem like an unaffordable luxury. This immediacy orientation makes the poor less able and less amenable to taking actions geared to preventing illness that might occur in the future—in such circumstances, that's not an easy concept to embrace.

In general, middle class families, which many say is a shrinking group, are able to meet the financial demands of everyday life, and may manage to have modest amounts of disposable income or savings. The orientation of the middle class accommodates both the present and the future. Since they are able to envision a life in the future, many are motivated to ensure that they remain as healthy as possible to enjoy that future. Disease prevention and health promotion are concepts they can embrace more easily than people in the poorer class. In recent years, however, the economic upheavals in the U.S. have pushed many middle class families into the throes of poverty as they lost their jobs, and consequently their homes to foreclosure. While the economy is slowly recovering, those who have remained unemployed over an extended period of time may be faced with a downward social mobility.

The wealthy, those in the highest rung of the social ladder, have an abundance of financial resources at their disposal that precludes them from having to be concerned about meeting their needs in the present or the future, as their wealth is often sufficient to last for generations. In addition to leaving an inheritance to loved ones, the wealthy are often interested in leaving a legacy to be remembered for. Again, because they envision a future, especially one with a purpose, the wealthy are interested in protecting, preserving, and prolonging the years of a healthy life for as long as they can. They often achieve this by incorporating both disease prevention and health-promotion practices into their lifestyle, and by accessing the best healthcare money can procure when they need it.

STAGES OF DISEASE PROGRESSION

As previously mentioned, epidemiologists have discovered that diseases, even those with a seemingly sudden onset like a heart attack, have been in the making for some time, having already passed through identifiable stages during their progression. Four such stages have been identified, beginning with one where the disease itself has not yet set in, but risk factors that predispose a person to the disease are present and lay the foundation for the impending disease. The duration of each of the four phases varies widely among diseases, the shortest being in infectious diseases and the longest being in chronic diseases, such as cancer, heart disease, and adult-onset diabetes. For the purpose of illustration, each of the four stages of the disease process is described here in the context of heart disease, which remains the number-one killer for both men and women in the U.S.

Susceptibility to Disease

With heart disease, a foundation for increased risk or susceptibility to it is laid via multiple factors, such as poor eating habits, unhealthy life-style choices—smoking tobacco, drinking beyond moderation, physical inactivity, inadequate rest and sleep, inability to manage stress effec-tively—and lastly a family history of heart disease. Family history as a risk factor is more indicative of the influence of learned and shared habits within a family than it is a genetic component, although the latter can and does play a part. It's not necessary for all the factors to be in play for the risk of the disease to increase. Some factors, smoking and being overweight for example, have a synergistic effect, meaning the two together exponentially increase the risk for heart disease, and don't merely equal the sum of the risk from each. Other risk factors that increase an individual's susceptibility to heart disease are having one or more other chronic diseases, such as diabetes or uncontrolled high blood pressure. It has long been known and documented that the risk of coronary heart disease among people with diabetes is significantly higher than it is among those without diabetes. In one meta-analysis of 37 prospective cohort studies of adult-onset diabetes and fatal coronary heart disease, published between 1966 and 2005, it was revealed that the average risk of coronary artery disease, the most common type of heart disease, was 3.5 times higher for those with diabetes than for those free of diabetes.[2] The risk was higher among women with diabe-tes than among men with the disease. Researchers explained that this greater risk among women with diabetes was due to the fact that they had more adverse cardiovascular-risk profiles, combined with possible disparities in treatment that favored men with diabetes. It should also be pointed out that no matter how strongly a particular risk factor is associated with a disease, that does not mean all individuals with that risk factor will necessarily develop the disease, nor does it mean those without the risk factor will not develop the disease. For example, some non-smokers do develop lung cancer, while some smokers never do. This seeming paradox is rooted in the *multiple causation* theory that disease is the result of multiple, interacting risk factors and not the result of any single cause. Nevertheless, exposure to one or more risk factors does increase the odds of developing the disease. In epidemiological parlance, this is referred to as *relative risk* (RR). If, for example, smokers are said to have an RR of 10.0 for lung cancer, it means they are ten times more likely to develop lung cancer than non-smokers. While the pathological changes in the body have not yet occurred in the susceptibility phase, the confluence of multiple risk factors creates the perfect storm to enable the next phase of the disease progression to begin, when abnormal changes in the tissues begin to take place.

Pre-Symptomatic or Pre-Clinical Disease

The second phase in the progression of a disease begins when there is still no outward manifestation of the disease in the form of *signs,* such as an elevated blood pressure or body temperature, and the person feels no symptoms, such as pain or other discomfort, swelling, or difficulty breathing. However, by this stage the disease has set in and has begun to cause abnormal changes in the body that can be detected by diagnostic tests and procedures. These include testing blood or other body fluids for the presence of disease-causing organisms or chemicals, abnormal elevation or suppression of the normal levels of biochemical values, examining tissue samples for abnormal changes, and X-rays and other radiological imaging for skeletal and other structural abnormalities. The interventions in the pre-symptomatic stage are aimed at reducing or reversing the abnormal changes set in motion by the early disease process in order to minimize its impact on the body.

In the heart-disease example used above, the blood test might show elevated levels of total cholesterol as well as the LDL or the bad cholesterol, and the triglycerides. An electrocardiogram (EKG) might show abnormalities in the functioning of the heart. These procedures, coupled with the clinical judgment of the healthcare provider, aid in early diagnosis and appropriate intervention that often prove effective in keeping the disease from progressing to the next, more advanced state. The rate of disease progression is accelerated in people with other risk factors, such as hypertension, tobacco smoking, type-2 diabetes, obesity, and a genetic predisposition.

The Symptomatic or Clinical Stage

The third phase in disease progression, the symptomatic, or clinical stage, is so called because the disease has progressed to a state where it manifests in *signs* that a clinician can detect and may associate with a disease, as well as *symptoms* the affected individual is able to experience and describe. This is most often when people seek intervention and come in contact with a healthcare provider. In the case of heart disease, the affected person may begin to experience such symptoms as chest pain, difficulty breathing during mild or moderate exertion, or swelling of the feet and lower legs due to fluid retention. If the symptoms are severe enough, the individual could arrive in the emergency room and subsequently hospitalized. Most often, however, the individual will seek intervention before then and will be diagnosed and treated for symptoms that don't require emergency care or hospitalization. A variety of drugs are available to treat the symptoms and manage the disease that could become chronic. The healthcare provider may also recommend lifestyle changes to arrest or slow down progression of the disease.

The Disability Stage

The fourth and final phase in disease progression is called the stage of disability. The label is somewhat misleading because not all diseases leave the person with a lasting disability. Some diseases are self-resolving, meaning they run their course and completely clear up without the person having any temporary or permanent disability of any kind. There are, however, other disease conditions that, after the acute phase has passed, leave the affected individual with lasting, in some cases permanent, disability or loss of function. This loss of function can take many forms for those affected, including limitation of physical activities as well as altered psychological and social functions. For the individual, his or her family, and society, the duration and extent of disability resulting from a disease, especially from a chronic illness, has many costs associated with it. Finally, there are some disease conditions for which there is no effective treatment other than temporary relief of symptoms that progress rapidly, and ultimately result in death. In heart disease, the person could have one or more heart attacks, requiring urgent medical intervention to stabilize and transport him or her to a hospital. A heart attack often results from a lack of blood supply to the heart caused by one or more blocked arteries. In the past, death due to a heart attack was more common, but with better drugs and medical devices, plus improved training of the emergency rescue personnel, many more lives are being saved today.

You might say, since people are living longer than ever before, they ultimately have to die of something. True, no one is meant to live forever, but the degenerative diseases mentioned here cause a lot of misery—physical, emotional, and economic—over an extended period of time before they eventually lead to death. By preventing, or in some cases postponing, the development of disease, it's possible to preserve the quality life by living disease-free for many years. The evolving and expanding knowledge about the interacting multiple factors that eventually cause diseases, especially those that cause high rates of illness and death, offers opportunities for prevention at every stage of the disease progression described above, including before the disease ever sets in. Needless to say, disease prevention requires investment on many fronts—the individual, the society, and the healthcare industry. Most importantly, at the individual level, it requires a reframing of the thinking about the role lifestyle choices play in averting or stopping the disease in its early stages, and at the societal level, it requires recognition of the importance of disease prevention in improving public health. The health care industry too needs to champion the cause of disease prevention with the same zeal and competence as it does with the treatment of disease once it sets in.

2

The Role of Exposure to Risks in Disease Causation

In the previous chapter, the concept of disease as the culmination of a process involving the interplay of multiple risk factors over a long period of time was introduced. In this chapter, the connection between risk exposure and the development of disease is explored.

The word *risk* used in the context of health and disease is defined as the exposure to conditions or behaviors associated with a higher probability that disease, injury, or death could occur at some point in life. For example, decades-long research has shown that a person who smokes has a much higher probability of developing lung cancer in his or her lifetime than a non-smoker. This statement does not imply that every smoker is certain to develop lung cancer or that a non-smoker would never develop the disease. The explanation for this lies in the fact that disease causation is multifactorial, and not the result of any single factor, no matter how strong a role that factor plays. There are many recognized risk factors associated with an increased risk for chronic diseases. For example, if an individual is overweight and smokes, the risk for heart disease is not simply the sum of the risk from overweight and smoking, but is far greater because of the combined effects of interaction between the two factors, referred to as the synergistic effect, described earlier. Add to this mix, habitual physical inactivity, which is also associated with an increased risk for heart disease, and the synergistic effects of the three combined factors balloon the risk manifold. For this reason, successful prevention of any chronic disease requires taking into consideration the combined effects of multiple risk factors, and the use of a multipronged approach to prevent, stop, or minimize exposure to all the relevant risk factors.

Not all factors associated with an increased risk for disease are modifiable. Modifiable risk factors include those you can avoid or minimize your exposure to, such as poor eating habits, physical inactivity, smoking, excessive alcohol consumption, and ineffective stress management, all of which increase the probability of developing one or more chronic diseases. Non-modifiable risk factors are those you have little control over being exposed to, such as your age, sex, race, ethnicity, and genetic make-up. All of these play a role in increasing your chances of developing such diseases as age-related dementia, breast cancer in women, sickle-cell anemia in African-Americans, and Tay-Sachs disease in Ashkenazi Jews of Eastern European ancestry.

In later chapters, the association between the risk of exposure to specific agents or behaviors and the corresponding increase in risk for certain chronic diseases will be discussed in greater detail.

ASSESSMENT OF RISK FROM EXPOSURE

In this chapter, we will examine the general concepts related to the link between risk exposure and the probability of developing a disease, and how that knowledge can be brought to bear on risk reduction and ultimately disease prevention. Epidemiologists and other public health professionals are interested in knowing who is most at risk for a given disease, so they can target their prevention and early-detection efforts toward those most vulnerable for developing a disease. For example, they want to know what is the probability of developing lung cancer among smokers relative to non-smokers, and if there are variations in smoking rates among subgroups of a population.

The probability rates of developing a particular disease are based on the incidence and prevalence data collected from national and international records on actual disease rates for the entire population, as well as for subgroups such as those exposed to the presumed risk factor and those who are not. The rate of occurrence of new cases of a disease, called the *incidence rate,* is calculated by dividing the number of new cases of a disease in a population over a specified period, like a year, divided by the number of people at risk for the disease. These could be the entire population in a geographic region unless it is known that a subgroup is not at risk by virtue of factors like age or gender. The incidence rate is also computed for subgroups exposed to a risk factor, like lung cancer among smokers for example, relative to those not exposed (non-smokers). The ratio of the rates between two groups being compared is called the *relative risk.* Let us say the incidence rate of lung cancer among smokers is 500 per 100,000 and the corresponding rate among non-smokers is 50 per 100,000. The risk ratio of lung cancer among smokers to non-smokers is 10:1, which translates to *smokers being ten times more at risk* of developing lung cancer than non-smokers. This is a hypothetical scenario, and in reality the ratio has been reported to be even higher. Another way the epidemiologists quantify the added risk of exposure to a known or suspected risk factor and the disease is by subtracting the incidence rate of the disease among the non-exposed from the incidence rate among the exposed. This difference in rates is called the *attributable risk,* signifying that the excess risk among the exposed can be attributed to a specific factor, like smoking in the example above. It is generally recognized that the higher these two numbers, *relative risk* and *attributable risk,* the greater the harm of exposure to the particular risk factor.

CAUSE OR COINCIDENCE?

It is important to know if an observed association between exposure to a specific factor and a disease is causal or a mere coincidence. This is easy enough to determine in such illnesses as infectious diseases where the cause is attributable to a single microbe, or in the case of a non-infectious disease where the cause can be determined by specific diagnostic tests. Chronic diseases, however, are caused by multiple, interacting factors that have been in play for years or decades. Epidemiologists have made it their mission to develop methods to effectively untangle associations between a suspected risk factor and disease prevalence. Skeptics in the healthcare field and beyond have challenged claims that the observed association between risk exposure and disease is necessarily causal. One such challenge came from the tobacco industry, insisting for years, that cigarette smoking did not cause lung cancer because non-smokers also developed lung cancer. While, due to their training and temperament, it is characteristic of the medical and scientific community not to accept any assertion that leaves room for rival explanations, the objections from the tobacco companies were largely profit-driven. To respond to these challenges, epidemiologists developed certain criteria for determining what constitutes a causal link between exposure and disease.

Here are five criteria proposed by epidemiologists to definitively determine a link between risk exposure and disease development.[1]

1. The association between exposure to a risk factor and the disease, positive or negative, should be strong, as evidenced by the relative risk (risk ratio), and attributable risk, both of which refer to the difference in the rate of disease among the exposed vs. the non-exposed. The larger the numbers of these two rates the greater the likelihood that the association is causal.

2. A second criterion is also related to the strength of the association between the risk exposure and the disease, and is evaluated by a corresponding incremental rise or fall in the two, referred to as a *dose-response* relationship. The presence of such a relationship demonstrates that the association is not merely due to chance or bias. If smoking is a cause of lung cancer, then within the smoking population those who smoke more should be at a higher risk of developing the disease than those who smoke less. The subsequent fact that the risk for lung cancer among smokers is reduced when they stop smoking also attests to the causal link between smoking and lung cancer.

3. The association between exposure and disease should endure across settings and different groups within the population. In other words, studies done in different geographic regions, different age, sex, race, ethnic, and socioeconomic groups, and even across different

methods of studies, such as retrospective (going back in time), as well as prospective (going forward in time) should yield results that consistently point in the same direction.

4. The presumed cause (exposure to a risk factor) should precede the disease and not the reverse. Given that chronic diseases, generally, have a long latency period, this criterion is not as easy to meet. Nevertheless, it should be ascertained that the exposure predated the disease, no matter the length of time between the two occurrences.

5. A fifth criterion is called *specificity* and states that one risk factor is specific to one disease. Although relevant in infectious diseases, this criterion does not actually apply to chronic diseases, as several chronic diseases can share many of the same risk factors, including overweight and obesity, physical inactivity, and smoking, which are all risk factors for cardiovascular diseases, type-2 diabetes, and some types of cancer.

By now it has been established that, although one factor may play a key role in the development of disease—smoking and lung cancer, for instance—chronic diseases are not caused by any single agent or factor, but by a combination of factors. Most chronic diseases have a long latency period between exposure to risk and the manifestation of disease. Several decades may go by before a smoker develops lung cancer that is attributable to smoking, and in the interim, the person may even have stopped smoking, but the foundation for later disease would already have been laid during the years of smoking, and revealed years later in the form of a malignant tumor. A similar scenario exists with other chronic diseases, such as heart disease and diabetes. A diagnosis of the disease during a routine visit to a healthcare provider, or in the emergency room, as might happen in the case of a heart attack that may seem sudden and dramatic (as well as traumatic to the individual and the family), but it is simply the culmination of a disease process begun long before. The characteristic natural progression of a chronic disease (its *natural history*) provides opportunities for you and your healthcare provider to stop the disease before its onset, or barring that, to stop it in its tracks through early detection and intervention.

Evidence-based information about what factors predispose a person to a particular disease is available, abundantly in some cases, thanks to extensive research in this area for decades, and even a century with respect to some diseases like heart disease. Knowing what risk factors are associated with a chronic disease, coupled with established evidence-based protocols for early detection, makes disease prevention during the various stages of progression, including before it ever sets in, not only possible, but also imperative.

3

Lifestyle Choices and the Connection to Chronic Diseases

Previously, the concept that disease, especially a chronic disease, is a process that spans a long period of time, beginning with the stage of susceptibility where there is no disease, but a foundation for it is laid, was described. That foundation consists of exposure to one or more recognized risk factors for the disease. Lifestyle choices, the type of diet you habitually eat, the level of physical activity you engage in, the weight you maintain, whether or not you smoke, drink alcohol in moderation or in excess, whether or not you get yourself at least seven hours of sleep in a twenty-four-hour period etc., fall under the category of modifiable risks (discussed in Chapter 2), whereas your age, sex, race, ethnicity, and genetics fall under the non-modifiable category. The steady increase in the rate of chronic diseases beginning in the second half of the twentieth century and reaching epidemic proportions in the twenty-first century has spurred an interest among epidemiologists and other researchers to look for causes of this unprecedented rise in their prevalence. Their search is underscored by the magnitude of the disease burden, and the skyrocketing costs of treating chronic diseases. The ensuing research has yielded an extensive and continually growing evidence-based body of knowledge on the role that personal health behaviors embedded in our lifestyle play in increasing or decreasing the probability of developing one or more chronic diseases. People have come to recognize that it is personal choices and not providence that plays a hand in whether or not a chronic disease develops, and how early or late in life it develops.

In Part 3, the lifestyle choices that help promote your health and protect you from chronic diseases and associated premature death will be discussed in greater detail. Here the connection between selected lifestyle choices and later development of a chronic disease is examined from a conceptual aspect. A landmark study undertaken many years ago with Harvard University alumni best illustrates this connection.[1] The purpose of the study was to find out how lifestyle in the areas of physical activity and smoking correlated with mortality in men. In a questionnaire, researchers asked over 10,000 male alumni about their physical activity, cigarette smoking, blood pressure, and body weight between 1962 and 1966. Based on the results of this initial survey, those participants who reported any diagnosed chronic disease at the time were excluded from further participation. In 1977, the researchers sent a second questionnaire to the remainder of the participants to ascertain any changes in their physical activity level and other health practices since they were first surveyed. The men in the study were between the ages of forty-five and eighty-four. In both questionnaires, the men reported how many city blocks (or the equivalent) they walked daily, the sports or recreational activities they engaged in, and the number and length of times they engaged in them per week. According to the intensity and frequency of the activity, they categorized the participants as light or moderately vigorous based on kilocalories expended per week. Similarly, with respect to their smoking habits, they divided the men into three categories—men who smoked a pack (twenty cigarettes) a day, those who smoked less than a pack a day, and non-smokers. The men were followed for nine years forward, from 1977 through 1985. During the nine-year period, there were 476 deaths: 44 percent from cardiovascular diseases; 33 percent from cancer; 9 percent from trauma; and the remainder from natural or unknown causes. Researchers looked for associations between lifestyle and deaths from all causes, as well as from individual causes. They found a pattern of an inverse relationship between the levels of physical activity and the risk of premature death from any cause. A lower death rate was associated with all levels of physical activity, such as regular walking, stair climbing, and playing a moderately vigorous sport. Incremental benefits of a lower death rate were seen in all but light physical activity—golf, walking for pleasure, gardening, housework, and carpentry. The moderately vigorous sports activities included swimming, tennis, squash, racquetball, handball, and jogging or running. In this study, the relative risk of death among sedentary men relative to active men (at a moderate level of activity) was 1.25. Since relative risk is actually a ratio, this translates into 125 deaths among the sedentary men for every 100 deaths among the active men in this study. This is quite a significant finding about the power of physical activity, even of moderate intensity, to lower the risk of premature death. It should be noted that in order to isolate the effects of physical activity on the death rate, the researchers made sure that all other personal characteristics, including smoking, that could possibly have a confounding effect on the association were on par or were adjusted statistically to remove their effect.

Smoking had an even more dramatic effect on premature death with a relative risk of 1.87, reflecting 187 deaths among smokers for every 100 deaths among non-smokers, the excess deaths attributable to smoking alone, everything else being equal. Men who stopped smoking prior to the study had a 41-percent lower death rate than those still smoking, but still did not come close to the death rate achieved among non-smokers—yet another powerful message about a lifestyle choice with serious negative health consequences. The risk of death from all causes was higher for overweight men than for those of normal weight who had a 23-percent lower risk of death. The overweight and obesity problem is one that has been increasing exponentially in the general population worldwide, and has reached epidemic proportions, along with its companion chronic diseases, in the U.S.

During the nine-year follow-up period, there were 130 deaths from diagnosed coronary heart disease (CHD). Again, there were consistently more of these deaths among the less active, the overweight, and the smokers. For example, men who engaged in moderately vigorous activity at the time of the study had a 41-percent lower death rate from CHD than sedentary men. An incremental up or down difference was seen in all three lifestyle-associated death rates from coronary heart disease—physical activity, body weight, and smoking. The researchers point out that specific lifestyle characteristics—physical activity of at least moderate intensity, maintaining normal weight, and not smoking, are all beneficial not only in extending life, but also in extending healthy years with lower rates of disease. The findings of this study are consistent with other studies done both prior to and following this study. The researchers also pointed out that their findings are consistent with their own study of former varsity athletes, which showed that athletes who discontinued their sports activities had higher rates of disease and death than their teammates who continued vigorous physical activity.

The purpose of describing the above study is not to assert that a single study, especially one done on a select group, provides irrefutable evidence to generalize from, but simply to offer it as a testimony, not only to the presence of a connection between lifestyle choices, disease, and death, particularly from chronic diseases, but also to the strength of that connection. The incremental differences in rates of disease and death from all causes, as well as from specific chronic disease found in the study, attest to the strength of the connection.

Up to this point, the concept of disease as a culmination of risk factors, often over a long period of time, has been explored. From decades of research and the corroborating evidence generated as a result, it is known that a majority of people who develop a particular chronic disease, such as heart disease, share exposure to certain risk factors with other chronic diseases. These common risk factors include an unhealthy diet, physical inactivity, smoking tobacco, overweight and obesity, chronic unmanaged stress, a family history of the disease, and genetic pre-disposition to a disease. While not all of these risks are modifiable, it is helpful to know about the non-modifiable risks, such as a genetic pre-disposition to a disease, and be able to make informed choices to avoid or minimize its impact.

Chapters 4 through 7 in Part 2 of the book will address each of the major chronic illnesses—cardiovascular diseases (CVD), type-2 diabetes, cancer, and obesity. In each case, attention will be focused on the known risk factors associated with the disease, the pathway to the development and progression of disease (*natural history of disease*), and the corresponding pathological changes in the body. Opportunities for preventing these diseases before they set in or stopping them in their tracks through early detection and appropriate intervention, along with cultivation of positive health behaviors, will be explored.

PART 2

The Impact of Killer Chronic Diseases on Health

The chapters in this section of the book are devoted to describing the individual chronic diseases that are taking a toll on public health, with a focus on preventing and/or stopping them in their tracks through early detection and intervention to achieve a healthy longevity. Each of the chapters also contains case histories from one of the author's medical practice to illustrate the impact of exposure to risk factors on the development and progression of different chronic diseases, including the harm a delay in their diagnosis and treatment may cause, and conversely the health benefits that early detection and timely intervention confer on the individual.

4

Cardiovascular Diseases

The term cardiovascular diseases (CVD) encompass diseases of the heart and blood vessels. They are thus grouped for several reasons, but primarily because the body organs and systems affected by the diseases are anatomically and physiologically inter-connected, and the diseases share common risk factors. Heart disease continues to be the number-one cause of death among both men and women in the U.S. and worldwide, despite a steady decline in incidence in recent decades. According to an American Heart Association's 2013 report, between 2001 and 2011 alone, the death rate attributable to CVDs declined by nearly 31 percent.[1] Yet according to a 2015 report by the Centers for Disease Control and Prevention, every year over 610,000 people still die of heart disease in the United States, and about three quarters of a million people have a heart attack; nearly a third of these happen in people who have already had one or more prior heart attacks.

Susceptibility to CVD begins with exposure to one or more of the risk factors associated with this group of diseases, and escalates if the exposure continues over an extended period of time. When there is more than one risk factor involved, their synergistic effect (combined effect larger than the sum of individual factors) compounds the impact, and accelerates the progress of pathological changes in the body. For example, when an individual is overweight or obese and also smokes, the combined effect of these two risk factors is greater than the sum of the two factors individually in increasing the susceptibility to a cardiovascular disease. Having one or more other chronic diseases such as type-2 diabetes, technically referred to as co-morbid-ities or multi-morbidity, also significantly increases the susceptibility to a cardiovascular disease.

The death rate (deaths per 100,000 population per year) from heart disease is highest among black men, followed by white men and black women, and lastly by white women.[2] Despite a steady decline in the death rate from cardiovascular diseases in the past several decades as noted above, the burden from this group of diseases on both the individual and society, in terms of years of life lost, diminished quality of life, lost productivity, and healthcare costs, remains high. Known risk factors for cardiovascular diseases are multiple, and synergistic, resulting in a larger combined total effect.

The American Heart Association (AHA) defines cardiovascular health for adults twenty years of age and older as, not just the absence of a clinically determined cardiovascular disease, but as a simultaneous presence of four specific health behaviors, and three specific blood-test values in the normal range without the aid of treatment. The health behaviors include a lean body mass, abstinence from smoking, participation in regular physical activity, and eating a healthy diet. The desired blood-test values in the normal range are the total cholesterol, fasting blood sugar, and blood pressure.[3] These criteria have long been associated with a reduced risk for cardiovascular diseases, as well as other chronic diseases, such as type-2 diabetes, kidney failure, and certain types of cancer. In recent years, the AHA has set the ambitious goals of achieving a 20 percent improvement in the cardiovascular health of all Americans by the year 2020, and a 20 percent reduction in deaths from cardiovascular diseases by then. Achievement of these goals will require a buy-in and efforts by individuals, families, and soci-ety to invest in prevention as well as introduction and implementation of meaningful legislation by local, state, and federal governments in support of the goal.

CORONARY ARTERY DISEASE (CAD)

For nearly a century, coronary artery disease, the most common type of heart disease, has been studied to determine the risk factors that ultimately lead to the disease. The evidence gathered points to a strong link between CAD and an unhealthy diet, obesity, smoking, physical inactivity, alcohol consumption beyond moderation, and a family history of the disease (suggestive of a genetic pre-disposition). For a long time the dietary intake of cholesterol (fat) was believed to be the main culprit because cholesterol in the blood leads to plaque buildup in the arteries, causing them to harden (*atherosclerosis*) and restrict blood flow to the heart. This theory was supported by evidence from cross-cultural studies that revealed corresponding differences in diet and coronary artery disease. As far back as 1916, the Dutch physician De Langen compared cholesterol levels of the Dutch immigrants in the former Dutch East Indies with those of the native Javanese, and noted that the levels in the immigrant Dutch were nearly twice as that of the locals.[4] De Langen published an article proclaiming that the differences in cholesterol levels of the two groups were attributable to differences in their diet.

Three decades later, in 1948, the U.S. Public Health Service and researchers at The Harvard School of Public Health launched the Framingham Heart Study in Massachusetts that lasted for nearly 30 years.[5] This study became known worldwide as a landmark study for the strength of its methodology (a prospective cohort study), as well as its broad scope, and it laid the foundation for future epidemiological research on cardiovascular and other chronic diseases. The researchers of the study are credited with introducing the term *risk factor* into the medical lexicon and contributing to cardiac risk scoring in later years. This landmark study identified several risk factors for heart disease, and revealed the disease was more prevalent among smokers and those with high cholesterol levels, high blood pressure, low levels of physical activity, and those who are overweight or obese.

Ancel Keys and coworkers studied dietary cholesterol and death rates in the 1950s in the United States, Japan, and Northern and Southern Europe.[6] Their study, known as *The Seven Countries Study* as the research spanned seven countries, involved more than 11,500 men aged forty to fifty-nine years old who were free from disease at the start of the study and were followed twenty-five years into the future. The results showed that cholesterol levels were high among men in the United States and Finland, and low in Japan and Southern Europe. The research team also noted large differences in the rates of coronary artery disease that corresponded to differences in the dietary patterns of participants. These early studies emphasized the role of diet in elevating blood cholesterol levels, and ultimately causing coronary artery disease and eventual death. Diets consisting of more animal foods, with the exception of fish, were found to be associated with higher death rates, and diets consisting of more plant-based foods corresponded to lower death rates from the disease. Based on their findings, researchers noted that cross-cultural differences in diets could be associated with differences in average serum cholesterol levels, rates of heart disease, and deaths from heart disease in a population. They also observed that a higher ratio of monounsaturated fats (e.g. olive oil) to saturated fats—butter or lard—in the diet was especially protective, as it showed a lower death rate among the study's participants.

In the latter part of the twentieth century, research on fat metabolism revealed that total cholesterol was composed of three

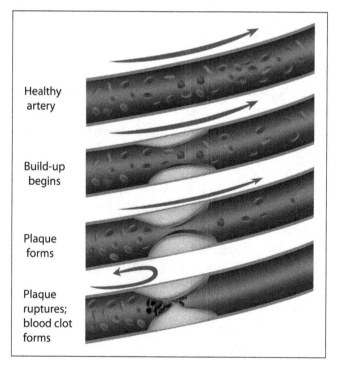

Healthy
artery

Build-up
begins

Plaque
forms

Plaque
ruptures;
blood clot
forms

Figure 1.
Stages of
Atherosclerosis

subcomponents—high-density lipoprotein or HDL, low-density lipoproteins or LDL, and triglycerides. Researchers also found that the
amount of LDL, often referred to as the bad cholesterol, in the blood
was most strongly related to the development of atherosclerosis and
eventual heart disease, and that the total cholesterol was less of a factor
in plaque buildup. It is now well known that cholesterol consists of
component particles or lipoproteins of varying densities—high, low,
and very low. The HDLs, often referred to as the good cholesterol,
consists primarily of protein and less of cholesterol and triglycerides.
The HDLs do not penetrate the walls of the arteries, and thus do not
contribute to plaque buildup, an attribute considered beneficial for
heart health. The Framingham heart study, mentioned earlier, demonstrated that people with high HDL levels had the lowest risk of developing coronary artery disease, and conversely those with the low levels
of HDL had a much greater risk. This protective effect of HDL is also
believed to come from its ability to remove excess cholesterol from
blood and transport it to the liver from where it enters the digestive
system and is eventually excreted. In addition, HDLs may play other
useful roles, such as promoting the health of the endothelium (the
lining of the blood and lymphatic vessels, heart, and other organs) by
reducing inflammation. The HDLs are increasingly being studied for
the development of new and more effective treatment modalities for
atherosclerotic cardiovascular disease.

The low-density lipoproteins (LDLs) consist mainly of cholesterol,
and the very-low-density lipoproteins (VLDLs) consist mainly of triglycerides. Both the LDLs and the VLDLs penetrate the walls of
arteries and are believed to be responsible for plaque formation that
builds up over time and results in atherosclerosis or hardening of the
arteries. The extent of *atherogenesis* (plaque formation) is determined
by both the amount and duration of the rise in the cholesterol levels, particularly the low-density lipoproteins (LDLs and VLDLs). A
higher than normal value of low- and very low-density lipoproteins
in the blood is considered a risk factor for heart disease due to their
artery-clogging properties. A significant amount of plaque buildup in
the arteries can result in narrowing of the lumen (known as *stenosis*)
and restricted blood flow to the heart, which can lead to such cardiac

events as a heart attack. Saturated fats in the diet, mostly consumed through animal products (with the exception of fish), and trans fats, taken in through eating foods containing hydrogenated oils (e.g. shortening) commonly used in baked goods, and many processed foods, can raise both the LDL cholesterol and triglyceride levels that pose a risk for heart disease.

More recently, the amount of added sugar in the diet has been recognized as the single most important cause of obesity and type-2 diabetes worldwide, both of which also pose a significant risk for heart disease.[7] Sugar is believed to play a role in fat metabolism, especially in raising serum triglycerides that are the stored form of sugars. Acknowledging the link between sugar consumption and weight gain, the American Heart Association has recommended that women consume no more than 100 kilocalories (equal to 6 teaspoons of table sugar, honey, or corn syrup), and men no more than 150 kilocalories (9 teaspoons) from sugar in any form per day.

It has long been known that atherosclerosis is an inflammatory disease of the inner layer of the arterial wall, caused by the accumulation of cholesterol-carrying LDL and VLDL particles. This inflammatory process sets a vicious circle in motion in the arterial lining, which leads to a slow progression of lesions. Cholesterol (primarily LDL and VLDL) is the main ingredient, and inflammation is the process by which plaque is formed, and culminates in hardening of the arteries.[8] Epidemiological studies have demonstrated that cardiovascular risk factors are identifiable in childhood and are predictive of risk for coronary artery disease in adulthood. The first signs of fat deposits, called fatty streaks, have been found in the lining of major blood vessels in children as young as 10 years of age. If exposure to one or more of the risk factors is not addressed at a young age, over time these fatty streaks may progress to plaque buildup, causing thickening of the arteries and narrowing of the lumen, setting the stage for the development of cardiovascular disease (see Figure 1 on page 38). Pathology studies done from autopsies performed after an unexpected death of children and young adults have shown both the presence and extent of atherosclerotic lesions associated with established risk factors in adults. A longitudinal cohort study in a semirural black and white community in Bogalusa, Louisiana that has come to be known as the Bogalusa Heart Study, has also lent much credence to this claim.[9] Between September 1973 and December 1996, researchers followed children ages four to seventeen to their adult ages of eighteen to thirty-eight years, to examine the association between the thickness of the carotid artery wall, a reliable and frequently used measure of atherosclerosis in young adults, and the traditional cardiovascular risk factors. The study provided serial observations from childhood to young adulthood that made it possible to measure the cumulative burden of risk factors since childhood. Based on their findings, the researchers concluded that childhood measures of LDL cholesterol level and body mass index (BMI) reliably predicted carotid artery thickness in young adults. These observations from a community-based cohort suggest that elevated LDL cholesterol and BMI levels are important risk factors early in life and may be predictive of eventual coronary artery disease risk. There is also now substantial scientific evidence that behaviors associated with risk factors in early life, including poor dietary habits, physical inactivity, and the use of tobacco, do set the stage for the later development of cardiovascular disease.

HYPERTENSION (ABNORMALLY HIGH BLOOD PRESSURE)

Hypertension is a disease of chronically elevated blood pressure, with abnormal physiological changes in the body that may not manifest as symptoms until the disease has advanced, a reason why this disease is referred to as the silent killer. Your blood pressure is simply the pressure (tension) exerted by the blood flow against the walls of the arteries. When you have your blood pressure measured, you are given two numbers—the upper *systolic* and the lower *diastolic.* Systole is the contraction phase of the heart's pumping cycle when the blood is forced out of the heart chambers for circulation throughout the body, and is a measure of resistance in the arteries. Diastole represents the reverse phase, when the heart muscle relaxes and dilates to receive the incoming blood, ready to be pumped throughout the body, and is a measure of the remaining arterial resistance during this phase. Although the guidelines for what constitutes normal blood pressure for different groups of people have changed slightly in recent years, it is generally defined as a systolic pressure equal to or less than 130 mm Hg (millimeters of mercury), and a diastolic pressure equal to or less than 85 mmHg in adults over the age of 18 years (to be read as 130/85 mmHg or less).

Your blood pressure is influenced by many factors:

- Your age, which affects the elasticity of the arterial walls

- Your weight

- Your level of fitness

- Smoking

- Stress level

- High salt intake, such as added table salt or salty snacks

- Medications you may be on for the treatment of one or more other diseases.

It is estimated that one in four American adults has high blood pressure, defined as systolic pressure of 140 mm Hg or greater, or a diastolic pressure of 90 mm Hg or greater.[10] An additional 45 million people are presumed to fall into the pre-hypertensive blood-pressure range of 130–139/80–89 mmHg. Elevated blood pressure is associated with a two to three times higher risk of developing heart failure, and a substantially higher risk of having a stroke or end-stage kidney disease. Blood pressures of 160/90 mm Hg or greater are associated with a risk for strokes, estimated at four times greater than for those with blood pressure in the normal range. Both the rates of incidence (new cases) and prevalence (total number of people living with the disease) of hypertension are increasing, and nearly a third of those with hypertension are estimated to be unaware that they have it. Only about a third (34 percent) of those who are diagnosed and on medication have it well controlled; the remaining show inadequate control or no control, often due to noncompliance with prescribed treatment. There are significant disparities in the prevalence of hypertension among the population groups. African-Americans develop elevated blood pressure at an earlier age, and have higher blood pressures on average. This leads to increased rates of strokes, heart-disease-related deaths, and a 4.2 times greater rate of end-stage kidney disease in this racial group. Hypertension is a largely preventable disease with healthy lifestyle choices. It is also an easily diagnosable and treatable disease, which, if achieved in the early stages, can prevent or thwart other, more serious cardiovascular diseases.

Stroke

A stroke, also known as a *cerebrovascular accident* or a *brain attack*, occurs when the blood supply to the brain is cut off (an *ischemic* stroke), or when a blood vessel bursts and bleeds into the brain (a *hemorrhagic* stroke). The majority (87 percent) of the strokes are of the ischemic type, caused by a cerebral infarction that occurs when a blood clot or a ruptured plaque results in blocked carotid or cerebral arteries. Without oxygen getting to them, the blocked arteries then cause brain cells to begin to die. High blood pressure, smoking, type-2 diabetes, and having had a previous cardiovascular event, increase a person's chances of having a stroke, which may result in permanent disability or death. Deaths from strokes have decreased dramatically and consistently in most countries during the last fifty to seventy-five years. This reduction in stroke-related deaths is due to steady improvements and innovations in the management of such diseases as type-2 diabetes that increase the risk of a stroke manifold; better diagnostic procedures that help detect and avert an impending stroke; and the early use of thrombolytic (anti-coagulant) drugs that can halt a stroke in its tracks and minimize the damage that might otherwise ensue. A stroke is still the third leading cause of death worldwide, and the fifth leading cause of death in the U.S. Each year, over 600,000 people in the U.S. have a stroke for the first time, and another 185,000 experience a subsequent stroke. According to the Centers for Disease Control and Prevention (CDC), in the year 2010, 2.6 percent of Americans eighteen years of age or older reported having had a stroke. It is projected that by 2030, an additional 4 million people will have had a stroke, increasing the number of people still living after a stroke by nearly 25 percent, 15–30 percent of them with some degree of permanent disability. The American Heart Association also estimates that in 2010 strokes cost about $53.9 billion in both direct and indirect costs in the United States. A stroke is more common in women than in men, among blacks than whites (the difference attributed to higher prevalence of chronically elevated blood pressure among blacks), and among those with lower income and lower educational attainment. One in seven, or about 15 percent of all strokes, are preceded by a transient ischemic attack (TIA). The TIA symptoms resemble those of a stroke, but resolve within a few hours to a day; hence TIA is sometimes referred to as a *mini stroke*. The risk factors for a TIA are the same as for a stroke, namely hardening of the arteries, intracranial and carotid (head and neck) arteries in particular, emboli (clots or masses of undissolved matter) to the brain, chronically elevated blood pressure, and type-2 diabetes. Studies have shown that the short-term risk of having a stroke after a TIA is substantial. Those who survive a TIA without a stroke beyond the initial high-risk period face a ten-year, 43-percent combined risk of having a stroke or other cardiovascular event.[10]

RISK FACTORS FOR CARDIOVASCULAR DISEASES

Unhealthy Diet

The amount of meat and saturated fat consumed in the U.S. clearly exceeds nutritional needs. The six major sources of saturated fats in the American diet are fatty meats, baked goods, cheese, milk, margarine, and butter. There is now substantial evidence that the absolute amount of dietary fat is less important than the type of fat in lowering the risk for chronic disease. Monounsaturated fats, such as those found in olive oil and other vegetable oils—canola and sunflower, for example—and polyunsaturated fats found in such plant foods as avocados, whole grains, and legumes are beneficial to health. Most saturated fats (from meats and full-fat dairy products) and trans fats (contained in shortening or in the hydrogenated oils used in baked goods) are known to be detrimental to health when consumed in large quantities. Research has shown that a ratio in favor of mono- and other poly unsaturated fats to saturated fats is more of a critical factor in preventing cardiovascular diseases than the absolute amounts of fats consumed.

One major diet and health study, conducted in 2009 by the National Institutes of Health (NIH) and the American Association of Retired Persons (AARP), examined how meat consumption affected mortality.[11,12] This large study of more than half a million men and women, between the ages of fifty and seventy-one years, evaluated the association between the consumption of three categories of meat and the overall death rate. The categories consisted of: red meat that included all cuts of beef and pork; white meat consisting of poultry and fish; and processed meats, such as bacon, sausage, luncheon meats, cold cuts, ham, and hot dogs. Based on their findings, the researchers concluded that those men who ate the most red meat had a 31-percent higher death rate than those who ate the least. Consumption of processed meat was associated with a 16-percent higher death rate, particularly significant because the participants consumed only 1.5 ounces of processed meat a day on average. A high intake of white meat (poultry and fish) was associated with a reduced rate of death among both men and women. The deaths from cardiovascular disease and cancer also followed the same pattern as total deaths in this study, and women were affected similarly as men. The results of the study held up even after the researchers took other health habits and risk factors among the participants into account. The findings of the NIH-AARP study, one of the largest of its kind, are also consistent with earlier studies that have established a strong link between red-meat consumption and chronic diseases like heart disease and cancer, colon cancer in particular.

The size of food portions in the U.S. has also been steadily increasing, both while eating at home and away from home. Nationally representative data from large food surveys conducted between 1977 and 1998 have all pointed to this trend.[13] During this period, portion sizes and energy intake for all key foods (except pizza) increased at all locations for the total U.S. population, aged two years and older. The portion sizes were found to vary by locations, with the largest increase in portions consumed at fast food restaurants and the smallest at other restaurants. Portion sizes of certain foods increased more than others.

Between 1977 and 1996, the average energy intake and portion size for salty snacks increased from 1.0 to 1.6 oz. (an increase of 93 kilo calories); the size of average soft drink increased from 13.1 oz. to 19.9 fl. oz. (nearly a 50 kcal increase per drink); and the average cheeseburger increased from 5.8 to 7.3 oz. (addition of 136 kcal). High-fat beef and pork, luncheon meat, and hotdog intake decreased slightly. Overall, Americans doubled their energy intake of French fries, hamburgers, cheeseburgers, and Mexican food, as well as sugared beverages, as a part of their meals in the twenty-year period. These trends provide a sense of how the proportion of energy sources for the average American changed for each age group, and translate into an increase in the total kilocalories consumed per day from 1,839–1,958 on average.

In the United States, chronic diseases, such as heart disease, cancer, and diabetes attributable to diet and lifestyle, represent by far the most serious threat to public health. Yet both are modifiable risk factors for a range of chronic diseases. According to the Centers for Disease Control and Prevention, in 2013–2014, nearly 71 percent of the U.S. adult population over the age of 20 years was overweight (more than 20 percent above normal weight) or obese (body mass index 30 or greater). A condition called *metabolic syndrome,* representing a cluster of cardiovascular risk factors triggered primarily by overweight and obesity, was formally added in 2001 to the International Classification of Diseases (ICD-9) as a category of disease. The growing awareness of the high costs imposed on society by the rising incidence of diet-related diseases provides a strong case for introduction of policies to promote a healthy diet, one that is diversified and balanced between foods of animal and plant origin and contains recommended amounts of macro and micro nutrients and fiber.

Diet, lifestyle, and lipoprotein (fat) metabolism, and the complex interactions between them, determine the development of cardiovascular disease. Due to their synergistic interaction, the combined effects of an unhealthy diet and such lifestyle factors as smoking and physical inactivity are larger than the sum of their independent effects in increasing a person's susceptibility to heart disease. Evidence from large, prospective cohort studies done more recently supports the assertion that a healthy diet and lifestyle, along with blood pressure in the normal range and low levels of serum cholesterol, are all associated with a low risk of coronary heart disease. Eating foods containing antioxidants has been credited with slowing the process of atherosclerosis by boosting the body's defense against the free radicals produced during the process of oxidation. Antioxidants counter the effects of oxidative stress and associated cell damage. They are found in many foods, such as brightly colored fruits and vegetables, grains, legumes, nuts, meats, poultry, and fish. Some known antioxidant powerhouses include (most) berries, broccoli, cantaloupes, carrots, collard greens, fish and shellfish, green peppers, kale, soybeans, squash, sweet potatoes, tomatoes, red wine, and all dry beans, especially the brightly colored ones like red and black beans. It is prudent to eat a variety of antioxidant-containing foods as part of your daily diet. Eating a well-diversified diet with a combination of foods in the right balance is now recognized as offering the most health benefits. This topic is explored in greater detail in chapter eight.

Smoking and Cardiovascular Diseases

According to the U.S. Surgeon General's report, the use of tobacco continues to be the single largest preventable cause of death and disease in the United States.[14] For over half a century now, studies that followed groups of smokers and non-smokers over long periods of time have shown a strong, graded relationship between cigarette smoking and coronary heart disease, among other conditions. One such study, sponsored by the British Medical Association, was done in England in 1951. It was conducted on a large volunteer sample of 34,440 male doctors concerning their smoking habits.[15] The participants were asked if they smoked cigarettes only, pipes or cigars (or both), or a combination including cigarettes (mixed smokers), the amount smoked, the duration, and, if relevant, the date of stopping. The doctors were followed for twenty years into the future, and the subsequent changes in their smoking habits, as well as the rates of death among smokers and non-smokers were recorded. Among cigarette smokers, the death rate for men under seventy years of age was twice that of lifelong non-smokers of comparable age. Among the participants over seventy years of age, the death rate among smokers was 1.5 times that of non-smokers. In all age groups, the death rate corresponded incrementally to the amount smoked—light, moderate, and heavy, the highest being among the heavy smokers and the lowest in light smokers. In every case, the death rate was higher in cigarette smokers than in those who smoked pipes or cigars, or both. Based on their findings, the researchers concluded that much of the excess mortality in cigarette smokers was attributable to the smoking habit, and that smoking caused death chiefly by heart disease, lung cancer, chronic obstructive lung disease, and various vascular diseases. The findings of this study about the association between smoking and chronic diseases were quite revealing, and although done more than six decades ago are quite relevant today. Smoking tobacco is a lifestyle choice and a significant risk factor for heart disease. Despite some progress achieved in this arena, a report by the Centers for Disease Control and Prevention states that one in five Americans still smokes, and more than three quarters of them smoke every day.[16] In 2009, nearly 1 in 5 students in grades 9 through 12 reported current tobacco use. In the U.S., exposure to secondhand smoke, even among children as young as four to eleven years of age, remains high. Research has shown that the percentage of smokers in a given population plays a role in explaining the differences in death rates from coronary artery disease. This is possibly due to the fact that unhealthy lifestyle choices tend to cluster. Studies done on smokers of all age and educational levels have revealed that smoking was associated with a higher consumption of all alcoholic beverages, and with less healthy dietary choices, compared to non-smokers. It is estimated that smoking-related illnesses cost the United States over $300 billion annually in medical expenses and lost productivity.[17]

A multinational study by the World Health Organization compared associations between lifestyle factors, such as smoking, biological risk factors (serum cholesterol, blood pressure, and body mass index), and coronary heart disease.[18] The study spanned twenty-one countries, most of them in Europe. The changes in major risk factors were analyzed in relation to changes in heart-disease rates among the populations. In men fifty-five to sixty-four years of age, the differences in serum cholesterol level alone accounted for 35 percent of the difference between fatal and non-fatal coronary events, such as heart attacks. When body mass index, smoking, and systolic blood pressure (the top number in blood-pressure reading) were also taken into account together, they accounted for half the population differences in heart attack rates. The *oxidation* of LDL cholesterol, and the elevation of triglycerides are believed to be the mechanisms by which smoking increases the risk for cardiovascular diseases. Both of these factors promote atherosclerosis (hardening of arteries) that is an underlying cause of all cardiovascular diseases, coronary artery disease in particular.

Physical Inactivity and Cardiovascular Diseases

Physical inactivity has long been recognized as a major modifiable risk factor for cardiovascular and other chronic diseases, on a par with smoking and poor dietary choices. Conversely, regular physical activity has been associated with a decreased risk of chronic diseases, cardiovascular diseases in particular. Evidence gathered from basic science, and epidemiological and clinical research suggests that habitual physical activity decreases the risk of fatal and nonfatal cardiovascular episodes, and that the benefits of regular physical activity outweigh its risks. Research has also established a direct association between physical inactivity and death from cardiovascular diseases, and has found that physical inactivity is an independent risk factor (regardless of exposure to other risk factors) for the development of coronary heart disease. The incidence of both acute myocardial infarction and sudden death has been reported to be highest in the habitually inactive or least physically active individuals.[19]

Exercise helps maintain body weight, prevents overweight and obesity, lowers blood pressure, improves metabolism, lowers the risk for diabetes, and counteracts atherosclerosis. In short, exercise contributes to cardiovascular health as well as overall health and wellbeing. Some have called exercise a miracle drug that can heap benefits on the total body and mind and contribute to healthy longevity. We might add that exercise is also the least expensive, sustainable therapy, with no side effects when done in moderation and with sensible precautions. Most of the beneficial effects of exercise to help prevent cardiovascular disease and death can be attained through moderately intense activity, such as thirty minutes of brisk walking on most days of the week, or preferably everyday. Like in the case of smoking, exercise also yields benefits in an incremental manner. A sedentary individual who becomes moderately active can derive the greatest potential benefit for reduced risk of death from cardiovascular diseases.

Findings of a meta-analysis (examining a group of similar studies) released in 2013 suggest that researchers and clinicians may be overly focused on a drug-based treatment of heart disease, and may be overlooking or downplaying the benefits of exercise in secondary prevention (early detection and timely treatment to halt the progression of disease) of coronary heart disease.[20] This study revealed that exercise and drug-based treatments might provide similar benefits in reducing death rates from heart disease and diabetes. The activity can be accrued through formal exercise training programs or leisure-time physical activities.

Recent research has also brought to light the fact that intensive multiple interventions, such as smoking cessation, blood-lipid reduction, weight control, and physical activity, significantly decreased the rate of progression and, in some cases, led to a lessened severity of atherosclerotic lesions in people with coronary disease. Those who remain sedentary have the highest risk of death from cardiovascular disease (when viewed alone), and from all causes. Conversely people remaining physically active or going from being sedentary to being physically active show the greatest decline in such risk. Questions about the minimum intensity needed for a cardio-protective benefit, and if risk decreases proportionately at higher intensities remain unsettled. Such questions have surfaced partly as a result of the recent changes in activity recommendations.[21]

THE NATURAL HISTORY (CHARACTERISTIC DISEASE PROGRESSION) OF CVD

The Susceptibility Phase

In an earlier section of the book, it was described how, during the susceptibility phase, the disease has not yet developed, but the foundation for it has been laid by exposure to certain factors that confluence to increase the likelihood of developing it. The role of several interacting factors that can cause CVD, such as an unhealthy diet, physical inactivity, and smoking, has also been described in some detail. The combined effect of two or more risk factors, like elevated levels of cholesterol (especially the LDL and VLDL components, triglycerides, smoking, and overweight or obesity), is greater than simply the sum of the individual factors, due to their synergy, and sets the stage for CVD by creating conditions that are optimal for development of *atherosclerosis* (hardening of the arteries), an underlying cause for CVD. This phase of disease development can often span many years and offers tremendous opportunities for stopping continued exposure to the risk factors and preventing the onset of the disease, and possibly reversing any damage already caused. This is called ***primary prevention***, and holds the most promise for preventing disease and protecting good health. The goal of primary prevention is pursued by all national and local public health organizations, as well as global entities like the World Health Organization (WHO), which are all committed to safeguarding the health of people everywhere. One program established in the U.S. toward this goal is the Million Hearts program, aimed at reducing the prevalence in the population of the leading risk factors for cardiovascular diseases.[22]

Asymptomatic Pre-Clinical Phase

When exposure to risk factors for CVD continues unchecked, pathological changes begin to take place in the body. However, at this early stage, the individual does not yet feel any symptoms and is unlikely to seek medical intervention, so the disease may remain undetected for some time while it continues to progress. A routine checkup along with recommended blood tests may reveal abnormal blood chemistry, such as elevated cholesterol levels, and triglycerides. This early, latent stage provides a window of opportunity for the medical provider and the patient to collaborate in stopping the disease in its tracks. Referred to as ***secondary prevention,*** this stage still holds promise for minimizing the ill effects of a full-blown disease through a multi-pronged approach to preventing or reducing further exposure to the relevant risk factors. If, for example, someone is overweight, smokes, and is physically inactive, the strategy could involve the person's stopping smoking, eating a healthier diet, and starting an exercise regimen. The healthcare provider would want to monitor the individual with follow-up visits at regular intervals, to ensure the disease is not progressing to the next, more advanced, stage.

The Clinical Disease Phase

The next stage in disease progression is often the result of continued exposure to one or more risk factors for CVD. During this phase, the disease-induced abnormal changes begin to manifest in the form of symptoms the affected individual may start to experience, and may seek relief by going to a doctor. The person may experience such telltale symptoms as shortness of breath, and chest pain or chest tightness when climbing stairs or engaging in similar exertion. The doctor may run a battery of diagnostic tests including an electrocardiogram (EKG) and certain blood tests. Based on the results of these tests, and the doctor's evaluation, the individual is placed on a therapeutic regimen. Concurrently, strategies to eliminate continued exposure to risk factors are put in place. It's never too late to halt exposure to risk factors as the benefits can be significant both in terms of stopping further progression of the disease, and even reversing existing damage, as recent studies have shown. In some cases, regression in the severity of atherosclerotic lesions in those with coronary disease has been reported. Results of pooled studies also reveal that people who start a regular exercise regimen after a cardiac episode like a myocardial infarction experience improved rates of survival.[23]

Severe Disease and Disability Phase

The final stage of cardiovascular disease may culminate in a sudden and dramatic event like a heart attack, which lands the person in an emergency room, and often leads to hospitalization. A set of therapies are initiated, including cardiac rehabilitation to not only aid in recovery from the acute episode but also steer the person toward a modified lifestyle to prevent or delay further episodes—as noted, death from a sudden cardiac event like a heart attack is not uncommon.

THE LESSON JAMES DID LEARN
FROM HIS HEART ATTACK

James is a sixty-two-year-old man who first came to see me in 2010 requesting a referral for a screening colonoscopy. He had not had a physical examination since his gallbladder was removed in 2008. His family history revealed that his father was diagnosed with hypertension, and had experienced a stroke and later died after a heart attack at the age of sixty-seven. His mother also had heart disease, but she lived to the age of ninety. James is 5′ 2″ tall, and weighed 182 pounds, with a body mass index (BMI) of 33 (30 and over is considered obese) when he came to see me. On the day of the visit his blood pressure was a normal 120/80 mm Hg. He had smoked cigarettes for thirty-five years before quitting in 2003, but he did not drink alcohol, and did not engage in any regular physical activity. An examination of his carotid blood vessels and heart and lung sounds did not signal anything abnormal. Although James was asked to schedule an appointment for a complete physical examination as soon as he could, I did not hear from him for the next three years. Then, I received a call from a local cardiologist that James had just suffered a major heart

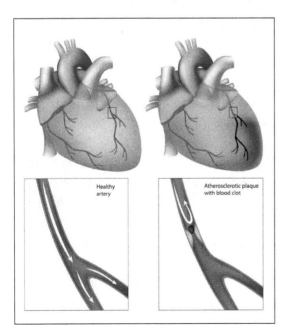

Figure 2. The Anatomy of a Heart Attack

attack and had undergone a successful cardiac catheterization, balloon angioplasty, and stent placement in one of his major coronary vessels.

During his hospitalization, James had several blood tests to check for any co-existing disease conditions, type-2 diabetes in particular. Sure enough, his fasting blood sugar was found to be above 200 mg/dL (normal range is 65 to 99), and his hemoglobin A1c was 10 percent (normal range is 4.5–5.6 percent), which meant that James had an average blood sugar level of at least 260 mg/dL over the previous three to four months. Both of these test values were strongly suggestive of type-2 diabetes. James also had an elevated low-density lipoprotein (LDL) of 148 mg/dl, more than twice the amount desired for someone with coronary artery disease and diabetes. His high-density lipoprotein (HDL) measured relatively low at 37 mg/dL (the desired level being 40 or greater for men). James was started on a medication regimen, appropriate for someone who'd just had a myocardial infarction, as well as to treat his newly discovered abnormally high blood-glucose levels. Upon his discharge from the hospital, James started making significant changes in his diet and increased his physical activity by walking regularly, which helped him lose a significant amount of weight fairly rapidly. His subsequent blood tests showed a definite improvement in his blood sugar and cholesterol levels.

James's case is a textbook illustration of how exposure to multiple risk factors leads to a chronic disease, sometimes more than one as in his case, and in the absence of timely intervention, progressed until culminating in a catastrophic event—the heart attack in his case. The risk factors that put James at increased risk of cardiovascular disease included his age, a family history of heart disease (both non-modifiable), a past smoking history, physical inactivity, and obesity (modifiable lifestyle choices). The multiple risk factors and their synergistic interplay continued unabated as he failed to have a timely assessment or intervention for his health problems that would have helped detect them in their early stages and prevent further progression to the catastrophic state, manifested as a heart attack.

To his credit, James took his heart attack as a wake-up call, and promptly made the needed diet and lifestyle changes that helped him lose weight and improve his blood-chemistry levels across the board. These actions should help him halt the progression of both his chronic diseases (heart disease and diabetes), avoid future complications, and improve his longevity. The moral of his story is that it is never too late to adopt healthier lifestyle choices, but the earlier you adopt them, the better it is for forestalling, or preventing the progression of disease to the next stage.

LUCKY LARRY AND HIS
MEDICAL TREATMENT TRIUMPHS

Larry is a seventy-year-old single (never married) man who has been my patient since 2010. He had a history of smoking a pack or more of cigarettes a day for forty years, drinking a six-pack of beer every day for many years, and not being physically active. In time, Larry developed chronic obstructive pulmonary disease (COPD) that manifested as a chronic cough and shortness of breath on exertion. His past medical history revealed that, in 2005, he quit smoking after a chest X-ray showed a mass in his right lower lung, and he underwent a lobectomy for non-small cell lung cancer followed by radiation and chemotherapy.

Four years later, in 2009, Larry was diagnosed with high blood pressure, and was prescribed a medication to control it, but he did not take the medicine regularly. In 2012, he had a stroke. Luckily, at the time Larry was with a friend at a ball game when he suddenly developed a weakness on his right side, slumped to that side, and lost his ability to speak. His friend notified the park authorities, and Larry was placed in an ambulance immediately and taken to the nearest hospital within minutes. After performing a CT scan and determining the type of stroke Larry had, he was given thrombolytic (anti-coagulation) therapy to dissolve the clot right in the emergency room. This timely intervention—the right treatment within three hours of onset is known to yield the best outcome for this type of stroke—ensured an excellent prognosis for Larry. He responded very well to the treatment and his right-sided weakness and speech impairment improved rapidly and resolved completely by the time he was discharged from the hospital.

While in the hospital, Larry developed aspiration pneumonia from food entering the wrong passage, and that exacerbated his COPD, requiring intubation (a breathing machine to help breathe). A few days later, his condition improved and he was taken off the breathing machine. During his recovery in the intensive care unit (ICU), Larry began to exhibit symptoms of alcohol withdrawal, which were brought under control and stabilized. Upon discharge he was advised to get treatment for his alcohol dependency.

Following his discharge, Larry started regularly taking his blood pressure and cholesterol medications, as well as a recommended baby aspirin. He started using his inhalers for his COPD properly, but did not cut down on his beer consumption.

Two years later, Larry developed an acid reflux problem that was not responding to medication, and he started experiencing difficulty swallowing and was frequently regurgitating mucous. An *esophagram* (a contrast x-ray of the esophagus) ordered by his pulmonologist showed a narrow, irregular segment in his upper esophagus. Larry was referred to a gastroenterologist who performed an endoscopy, and biopsied the suspicious looking segment of his esophagus. Based on the results of the biopsy, he was diagnosed with a squamous-cell carcinoma (cancer) of his upper esophagus. Larry completed four cycles of chemotherapy, and was subsequently referred to Stanford Hospital where he underwent tumor ablation with laser. He continues to be closely monitored to determine whether further therapy is needed.

Larry's lengthy medical history shows how a lifetime of unhealthy lifestyle choices involving cigarette smoking, excess alcohol consumption, and physical inactivity, can, over time, lead to multiple, concurrent chronic diseases—COPD, cancer, and hypertension, in his case. It also demonstrates how poor compliance with any recommended treatment regimen can lead to a catastrophic event that could have been avoided.

Larry happened to be at the right place at the right time when he had his stroke because being at a ball game in a major city certainly helped him get timely, appropriate intervention. His hospitalization for the stroke, followed by close monitoring for any ensuing related problems during office visits also led to the early discovery of his esophageal cancer and his alcohol dependency that might otherwise have gone undetected. In the end, Larry can give thanks to the advances in diagnosis and treatment for each of his ailments that are helping him stay alive and lead a fairly normal life. Not that long ago, given the multitude and severity of his health problems, Larry might have succumbed to a premature death.

5

Metabolic Syndrome, Pre-Diabetes, and Diabetes

The previous chapter discussed the fact that a great majority of people who develop a particular chronic disease, such as heart disease, share exposure to certain risk factors with those who might have another chronic disease, such as type-2 diabetes. That is to say, a set of risk factors working in concert can manifest in different disease conditions.

METABOLIC SYNDROME

A cluster of biochemical and physical conditions has often been known to precede the development of atherosclerotic cardiovascular disease and type-2 diabetes. Recognition of this clustering as foretelling of impending disease or diseases led clinicians and researchers to describe it as a syndrome that has come to be known as the *metabolic syndrome.* What is now called the metabolic syndrome, or the insulin-resistance syndrome, started with Gerald Reaven of Stanford University in the late 1980s when he described a cluster of abnormalities of metabolic origin that included obesity, insulin resistance, hypertension, impaired glucose tolerance or diabetes, *hyperinsulinemia* (excessive insulin in blood), elevated triglycerides, and a low level of high-density lipoprotein (HDL, the good cholesterol) in the blood. Reaven proposed that insulin resistance was at the center of this clustering, and that it is associated with increased risk for cardiovascular diseases and type-2 diabetes, and he called it *syndrome X*.[1] In later decades, a recognition that the cluster of conditions comprising the syndrome are all primarily metabolic in origin, syndrome X was renamed "metabolic syndrome," the term signifying that the condition is a composite of abnormal physiological conditions, metabolic in origin. Each of the conditions in the cluster is now widely recognized as not only being harmful in itself, but harmful together, portending an even more serious and possibly fatal atherosclerotic cardiovascular disease. The clustering in the syndrome is known to be the result of multiple factors, and not arising from any single cause.

Metabolic syndrome has also long been recognized as a multidimensional risk factor for cardiovascular disease (CVD), on the same footing as elevated low-density lipoprotein (LDL) cholesterol and is regarded a candidate for cardiovascular disease risk-reduction therapies. Although it is known that the clustering of metabolic abnormalities, characteristic of the syndrome, is the result of multiple factors, its root causes for the overwhelming majority of individuals are an unhealthy diet coupled with inadequate physical activity. This was best put in perspective by a group of researchers who applied a well-regarded statistical analysis technique to determine which of the factors played a role in causing the metabolic syndrome, and which ones contributed the most to it. Based on their analysis, they concluded that if the abnormalities related to metabolic syndrome were indeed spokes on a wheel with one central abnormality at the hub, that central factor would be obesity, which was found to be the common link between all the major facets of metabolic syndrome.[2]

Having metabolic syndrome nearly doubles the risk for cardiovascular disease, and raises the risk for type-2 diabetes by fivefold compared to those without the syndrome. The risks for both coronary heart disease and diabetes are greater from having metabolic syndrome than from obesity alone. For this reason, identifying those with the syndrome as early as possible in its development is regarded as useful in guiding both the treatment of individual conditions as well as preventing or arresting further damage, such as a plaque buildup in the arteries. There is evidence that a foundation for the conditions related to metabolic syndrome may even start in childhood or young adulthood, and build incrementally with age.[3]

Until fairly recently, classifying metabolic syndrome as a disease entity has been impeded by a lack of consensus on a uniform criteria for its diagnosis. According to guidelines used by the National Institutes of Health, a diagnosis of metabolic syndrome is made if three or more of the five traits described below are present in an individual.[4]

- Large waist circumference. This is defined as a waistline that measures at least 35 inches (89 centimeters) in women, and 40 inches (102 centimeters) in men.

- High triglyceride level. Having a triglyceride level of at least 150 mg/dL, (milligrams per deciliter) or receiving treatment for high triglycerides.

- Reduced high-density lipoprotein (HDL) cholesterol. This criterion is met if the HDL is less than 40 mg/dL in men, and less than 50 mg/dL in women, or if the individual is receiving treatment for low HDL.

- Increased blood pressure. This condition is met if blood pressure is at least 130/85 mm Hg or the person is being treated for high blood pressure.

- Elevated fasting blood sugar. Having a blood-sugar level of at least 100 mg/dL or being treated for diabetes.

Accumulated evidence shows that a significant segment of the adult population in industrialized countries develops metabolic syndrome. Based on the results of the Third National Health and Nutrition Examination Survey (NHANES), designed to assess the health and nutritional status of adults and children in the United States, it is estimated that on average about one in four adults in the U.S. has the syndrome.[5] The rate is about the same for white men and women, but among African Americans, women have about a 57 percent higher rate of prevalence than African-American men, and among Mexican Americans, women have about a 26 percent higher prevalence rate than Mexican-American men. The steadily increasing prevalence of obesity in the United States makes it likely that the incidence of metabolic syndrome will also keep rising.

Individuals with metabolic syndrome are at an increased risk for developing type-2 diabetes and cardiovascular disease and dying from cardiovascular disease, as well as from all causes. Insulin resistance, which is an underlying feature of metabolic syndrome, results in the body's inability to receive and utilize glucose for normal body functions. When this occurs, the body initially responds by stimulating the pancreas to secrete more insulin that results in what is known as *hyperinsulinemia* (excessive insulin in blood). For as long as this compensatory overproduction of insulin can be maintained, the body can continue to utilize glucose normally, but as insulin resistance worsens, the liver begins to produce glucose in increasing amounts and that leads to impaired glucose tolerance (IGT). At this stage, if the person's fasting blood glucose (after not eating or drinking liquids for at least eight hours) were to be measured, it would be at an abnormally high level. If the condition persists, a rise in triglycerides, a decrease in HDL cholesterol concentration in the blood, and a rise in blood pressure will often follow. All of these are known risk factors for cardiovascular diseases, coronary heart disease in particular.[6]

THE NATURAL HISTORY OF METABOLIC SYNDROME

The risk factors that increase susceptibility to metabolic syndrome are primarily lifestyle choices that contribute to overweight and obesity. Physical inactivity coupled with excessive caloric intake contributes significantly to the development of this syndrome. Weight loss, even of modest proportion, has proven very effective in decreasing the symptoms associated with the syndrome. Studies have shown that a loss of 7–10 percent of body weight is sufficient to result in improvements in waist circumference, levels of triglycerides, high-density-lipoprotein cholesterol, blood sugar, blood pressure, as well as in reducing abdominal fat.[7] Even this small a loss of weight, which can be achieved by incorporating exercise of moderate intensity for thirty minutes a day, has proven effective not only in stopping further progression of the syndrome, but also in helping to reverse abnormal physical and chemical values and return them to close to normal.

If exposure to known risk factors for metabolic syndrome continues unabated, then one or more of the five traits of metabolic syndrome listed above (under diagnosis of the syndrome) begin to take root. Clinical examination combined with blood tests may indeed signal the presence of the syndrome.

The next stage in metabolic syndrome is a clinical phase that requires therapeutic intervention involving one or more drugs, in addition to a modified diet and exercise. Given that the metabolic syndrome poses an increased risk for type-2 diabetes as well as cardiovascular diseases, it is critical to focus attention on controlling, even reversing, metabolic syndrome. If allowed to continue uncontrolled, the condition will likely lead to type-2 diabetes, or coronary artery disease, two chronic diseases with long-term detrimental effects on health and longevity. This underscores the importance of having metabolic syndrome treated to prevent diabetes, and cardiovascular diseases, including hypertension, chronic kidney disease, and stroke.[8]

PRE-DIABETES

Pre-diabetes is a condition that pre-stages type-2 diabetes. While it is not a certainty that all those diagnosed with pre-diabetes go on to have full-blown diabetes, those who do have it stand a much higher chance (4–7 times higher according to some estimates) of developing full-blown type-2 diabetes. According to The Centers for Disease Control and Prevention (CDC), there are millions of Americans (57 million as of 2011) who have pre-diabetes, and just 7.3 percent of them are aware that they have the condition.[9] Pre-diabetes also increases the risk of developing other life-threatening diseases, such as heart disease and stroke. A rapid progression of *atherogenesis* (development of arterial plaque), and an accompanying increase in the risk for coronary artery disease are commonly found in those diagnosed with pre-diabetes.

Most of the glucose in the body comes from the foods you eat, specifically foods that contain simple carbohydrates. During digestion, sugar enters the bloodstream, and with the help of insulin (a hormone secreted by the pancreas), it is absorbed into the body's cells to be used as energy. When you eat, your pancreas secretes insulin, and releases it into the bloodstream. As insulin in the blood circulates, it allows sugar to enter the cells, consequently lowering the amount of sugar in your bloodstream. As your blood-sugar level drops, so does the amount of insulin secreted by the pancreas. Pre-diabetes is a condition characterized by impaired glucose tolerance (IGT) or impaired fasting glucose (IFG), which indicate a higher than normal glucose level in the blood. If your fasting blood sugar level is over 100 mg/dL (normal range is 65-99mg/dL) but less than 126 mg/dL (126 or over is diabetes range) you are considered to have pre-diabetes. In pre-diabetes, the blood sugar level is not high enough to be classified as diabetes, but portends future diabetes if there is no intervention. As blood glucose levels continue to rise, your body may develop a state of insulin resistance, the body's compensatory mechanism to secrete and release more insulin into the blood. Over time, the pancreatic cells that produce insulin wear out and eventually die, and the pancreas becomes dysfunctional.

Causes of Pre-Diabetes

Pre-diabetes, like other chronic diseases, is a disease of many causes, not just one single cause. Although researchers have found a link between some genes and insulin resistance (a term also used to describe pre-diabetes), carrying excess body fat, especially abdominal fat, and physical inactivity seem to be significant factors in the development of pre-diabetes.

The Susceptibility Phase

Susceptibility to pre-diabetes begins with exposure to one or more of the following risk factors.

- Being overweight, with a body mass index (BMI) above 25

- Habitual physical inactivity

- Being forty-five years of age or older

- Having a family history of type-2 diabetes

- Being a member of these racial/ethnic groups: African-American,

Hispanic American, Native American, Asian-American, Pacific Islander

- Being a woman with a history of gestational diabetes and/or having given birth to a baby that weighed more than 9 pounds (4.1 kilograms)

- Being a woman with a history of polycystic ovary syndrome

- Being diagnosed with high blood pressure

- Having abnormal cholesterol levels, including high-density lipoprotein (HDL) cholesterol readings below 35 mg/dL or triglyceride levels above 250 mg/dL

Risk exposure to pre-diabetes may be intercepted by lifestyle modifications, including even a modest weight loss of 7 percent, through changes in diet and doing moderate intensity exercise for at least 150 minutes per week. This particular lifestyle modification has been reported to effectively bring down the risk by as much as 58 percent by reversing the blood glucose abnormality. Additionally, using medication to bring down blood-glucose levels has proven effective in reducing the risk of full-blown diabetes. [10,11]

Pre-Clinical, Latent Phase of Pre-Diabetes

Pre-diabetes screening is recommended for those exposed to one or more of the risk factors mentioned above. Two tests are commonly used to diagnose pre-diabetes:

- **Fasting Blood Glucose Test (FBG).** This test measures blood glucose the first thing in the morning, after fasting for at least eight hours the night before. A normal fasting blood-glucose level is less than 100 mg/dL. If your fasting blood glucose is between 100 to 125 mg/dL, you are likely in pre-diabetes state.

- **Oral Glucose Tolerance Test (OGTT).** This test measures blood glucose after fasting for at least eight hours, and again two hours later after drinking a sugar-rich drink. Two hours after the drink, normal blood glucose level should be below 140 mg/dL. In pre-diabetes, the two-hour blood-glucose level tends to be between 140 and 199 mg/dL. If this level rises to 200 mg/dL or above, it is indicative of diabetes.

The Expert Committee on the Diagnosis and Classification of Diabetes Mellitus of the American Diabetes Association takes the position that the fasting plasma glucose (FBG) is the preferred test, and recommends using it universally to test and diagnose diabetes because of its ease of administration, its convenience, acceptability by patients, and lower cost relative to the *oral glucose tolerance test.*[12]

The main physiological indicator, a red flag for the presence of pre-diabetes, is a blood-glucose level that shows impaired glucose tolerance, impaired fasting glucose, or both. Several national and international organizations, including the American Diabetes Association, that are dedicated to the prevention and management of diabetes recommend that pre-diabetes testing include the *glycated* hemoglobin (A1C) test.[13] This blood test indicates the average blood-sugar level for the previous sixty to ninety days. It measures the percentage of blood sugar attached to hemoglobin, the oxygen-carrying protein in red blood cells. The higher the blood-sugar levels, the higher the A1C level. An A1C level between 5.7–6.4 percent is considered indicative of a pre-diabetes state. A higher level on two separate tests is indicative of diabetes. Certain conditions, such as pregnancy or having an uncommon form of hemoglobin, can make the A1C test inaccurate, and should be considered when using the test. A1C test is regarded particularly useful for those who wish to confirm (or not) a diagnosis of pre-diabetes or diabetes.

After the Diagnosis of Pre-Diabetes

Once detected, the treatment for pre-diabetes is targeted at weight loss and increased physical activity, both of which have proven beneficial in preventing or delaying the transition to type-2 diabetes. Studies have also shown that, in some cases, blood-glucose levels return to their normal range. The diagnosis of pre-diabetes is reversible and provides a window of opportunity for averting full-blown type-2 diabetes. In people with pre-diabetes, modest weight loss and regular physical activity can help prevent or delay type-2 diabetes by up to 58 percent. Modest weight loss could mean 5–7 percent of body weight. For a person weighing 180 pounds, that's nine to twelve pounds; for a 200-pound person, it's eleven to fifteen pounds. Getting moderate-intensity physical activity, such as brisk walking, at least for 150 minutes a week is beneficial for not only reversing pre-diabetes, but for overall health by aiding in weight control. Programs for lifestyle change, offered through the National Diabetes Prevention Program and led by the Centers for Disease Control and Prevention (CDC), can help participants adopt the healthy habits needed to prevent type-2 diabetes. Without lifestyle changes to improve their health, 15–30 percent of the people with pre-diabetes are estimated to develop type-2 diabetes within five years of being diagnosed with pre-diabetes.[14]

DIABETES

Diabetes is a chronic, progressive disease with gradual loss of pancreatic function, often remaining undetected for a long time due to the body's compensatory capacity that keeps the disease latent and hidden. The term diabetes refers to a group of diseases in which the body does not produce or properly use insulin to convert sugar, starches, and other food into energy needed for daily life. There are three main types of diabetes.

Type-1 Diabetes

Type-1 diabetes develops when the body's autoimmune system attacks and destroys pancreatic beta cells that produce insulin needed to regulate blood glucose. This results in failure of the pancreas to produce insulin in sufficient quantities required by the body. Without the required insulin, the cells cannot get the sugar they need for energy, and too much sugar builds up in the blood. Type-1 diabetes starts when the pancreas stops making insulin. This disease usually occurs during childhood or adolescence, and accounts for less than 10 percent of all diagnosed diabetes cases. In order to survive, people with type-1 diabetes will need lifelong insulin therapy delivered by injection or a pump. There is ongoing research to explore alternative therapies, such as replacement of diseased pancreatic beta cells with healthy cells. Although the term is no longer used, this type of diabetes used to be called *juvenile-onset diabetes mellitus* simply because nearly three-quarters of cases occur by twenty years of age. Type-1 diabetes is not associated with increased body weight like its adult-onset counterpart, type-2 diabetes. However, diagnoses of type-2 diabetes in children and adolescents are also increasing in the U.S., more frequently among American Indians, African Americans, Hispanic/Latino Americans, and Asian/Pacific Islander Americans than other racial and ethnic groups.

Gestational Diabetes

Gestational diabetes occurs in women and is defined as glucose intolerance that is first detected during pregnancy. In the U.S., gestational diabetes is found in approximately 7 percent of all pregnancies.[15] Although gestational diabetes usually goes away after pregnancy, women who have had it are at an increased risk for later developing type-2 diabetes, and about a third of them do develop the disease ten to twenty years down the road. The condition occurs more frequently among African Americans, Hispanic/Latino Americans, and American Indians, obese women, and women with a family history of diabetes. Gestational diabetes requires treatment to optimize maternal blood glucose levels, and lessen the risk of complications in the infant.

Type-2 Diabetes

Type-2 diabetes, the most common form of the disease, usually occurs in people who are forty-five years of age or older, but due to widespread childhood obesity, it is now increasingly found in children and adolescents as well. It is a lifelong disease that happens when the body's cells can't use insulin effectively or the pancreas can't make enough insulin to keep up with the demand. As a result, the cells can't get the sugar they need, and sugar builds up in the blood. Over time, this extra sugar in the blood can damage eyes, heart, blood vessels, nerves, and kidneys. For individuals born in the United States, the lifetime risk of developing type-2 diabetes, according to a study by the Centers for Disease Control and Prevention (CDC), is estimated to be approximately two out of five in both men (40%) and women (39%).[16] For anyone diagnosed with the disease at age forty, long-term survival is reduced by twelve and a half years, and the quality of life is diminished for a much longer period. Insulin resistance combined with insufficient insulin production by the pancreas is believed to cause type-2 diabetes. The major risk factors include age (forty-five years and above), overweight (body mass index of 25 or higher), first-degree relative (parent, sibling) with diabetes, habitual physical inactivity, women with a history of gestational diabetes, and being identified as pre-diabetic with impaired fasting glucose (IFG) or impaired glucose tolerance (IGT). Being a member of a high-risk ethnic group (African American, Latino, Native American, Asian American, or Pacific Islander) also increases the odds of developing type-2 diabetes.

According to the National Diabetes Statistics Report of 2014, released by the Centers for Disease Control and Prevention (CDC), 29.1 million or 9.3 percent of American adults were estimated to have type-2 diabetes in 2012, 21.0 million of them diagnosed, with 8.1 million remaining undiagnosed. Among Americans sixty-five years of age or older, in the same year 11.2 million or 25.9 percent were estimated to have type 2 diabetes. Overall, type-2 diabetes is a statistically underrepresented disease because it can go undetected for a long time and many who have the disease don't know they have it. The rate of new cases itself is also on the rise in the U.S., owing to both an aging population and the rising incidence of overweight and obesity reaching epidemic proportions. The increase is also attributed to a rising incidence of type-2 diabetes among children and adolescents, for whom it had been a rare occurrence in the past. Worldwide more than 422 million adults between the ages of twenty and seventy-nine were estimated to have type-2 diabetes, in 2014, according to a World Health Organization (WHO) global report on diabetes. The prevalence of diabetes globally is reported to have quadrupled in the years since 1980.[17] The increase is expected to be more rapid in the developing countries, indicating a growing burden of diabetes that can primarily be attributed to the increasing overweight and obesity in those countries.

In the medical community, type-2 diabetes and cardiovascular diseases (CVD) often are seen as two sides of a coin. Type-2 diabetes has been rated equivalent to coronary heart disease in terms of its devastating effects on the body, and conversely, many who have established coronary heart disease also have diabetes or its pre-cursors. This makes it appropriate for the clinicians who treat these two major chronic illnesses to not only be vigilant about the possible co-existence of the two diseases, but also to direct their attention toward preventing these two major chronic diseases in the healthy population.

THE NATURAL HISTORY OF TYPE-2 DIABETES

The incidence of type-2 diabetes is on the rise, not only among adults, but also among children and adolescents for whom it had been a rare occurrence in the past. This emerging trend is being attributed, among other factors, to the growing incidence of overweight and obesity that have reached epidemic proportions among both adults and children in the U.S.

Susceptibility Phase

Both genetics and environmental factors, such as obesity and a lack of adequate physical activity, which are associated with metabolic syndrome, are believed to play a role in the cause of type-2 diabetes. The fact that even a modest weight loss brings a significant improvement across the board in blood chemistry associated with the onset of type-2 diabetes attests to the power of the association between overweight or obesity, physical inactivity and this disease. Sustained weight loss, coupled with regular physical activity may prevent or delay the development of type-2 diabetes, and even reverse the disease in its early phases.

In addition to overweight, obesity, and habitual physical inactivity, there are certain non-modifiable risk factors that also increase the likelihood of type-2 diabetes. These include a first-degree relative (parent or sibling) with diabetes, a history of gestational diabetes or giving birth to a baby weighing more than nine pounds, being a member of certain ethnic groups—African American, Hispanic American, Native American, Pacific Islander, and Asian American—and being older than forty-five years of age. Although these risk factors are considered non-modifiable, early detection of type-2 diabetes, through screening at a younger than normally recommended age, close monitoring, and early intervention by a healthcare provider all go a long way in preventing or delaying the onset of the disease, slowing its progression, and preventing the devastating vascular, neurological, and other complications of this disease.

Pre-Clinical or Latent Phase

One of the reasons for an underestimate of true prevalence of type-2 disease at any given time is the fact that diabetes can remain undetected for a long time, without any symptoms being manifested even though pathological changes may be taking place in the body. Many people with the disease are first diagnosed when they develop one of its potentially life-threatening complications, such as heart disease, vision problems, or neurological symptoms. Clinicians are attuned to the silent nature of diabetes and routinely screen individuals deemed at risk for the disease. The American Diabetes Association recommends testing individuals who meet the following criteria, as they fall into categories of increased risk for diabetes.[18]

- Having a first-degree relative (parent, sibling, child) with diabetes

- Women who delivered a baby weighing 9 lbs. or more, and/or were diagnosed with gestational diabetes

- Having an HDL level less than 35 mg/dL and/or a triglyceride level above 250 mg/dl

- Having blood pressure equal to or greater than 135/80 mm Hg. or being treated for hypertension

- Being a member of a high-risk ethnic population (e.g. African American, Latino, Native American, Asian American, Pacific Islander)

- Women with polycystic ovarian syndrome

- Having conditions associated with insulin resistance (e.g. obesity)

- Having a history of cardiovascular disease

- Having an A1C equal to or greater than 6.5 percent, impaired glucose tolerance, or impaired fasting glucose on prior testing;

- Physical inactivity

If one or more of the above-mentioned criteria apply to you or a loved one, it would be prudent to talk to a healthcare provider about getting screened for type-2 diabetes (*see* Chapter 9).

Clinical Stage of Diabetes

In this stage, the disease has advanced and symptoms have begun to manifest. The most common symptoms are frequent and excessive urination, and excessive thirst. Other symptoms include weight loss despite an increase in appetite, a lack of stamina, blurred vision, drowsiness, frequent bladder and skin infections, and vaginitis in women. In type-1 diabetes, the symptoms usually appear abruptly in a matter of weeks, if not days. In type-2 diabetes, however, the symptoms appear more gradually over months or years, making detection of the disease more difficult. The diagnosis is often made during routine screening or by accident when the individual sees a healthcare provider for some other health problem. The American Diabetes Association has established that the diagnosis of diabetes be based on one of the following criteria.[19]

1. A fasting plasma glucose (FPG) of 126 mg/dL or above on two separate occasions

2. A two-hour plasma glucose of 200 mg/dL or greater during a glucose tolerance test (OGTT)

3. An A1C (the glycated hemoglobin) of 6.5 percent or greater

4. A random blood plasma glucose of 200 mg/dL or greater in a person with symptoms of uncontrolled hyperglycemia.

There are a variety of methods currently available for treating both type-1 and type-2 diabetes. Healthcare providers determine the appropriateness of each based on the prevailing scientific evidence, the individual circumstances, and the person's preference.

The Pathophysiology (altered physiological processes) of Type-2 Diabetes

Pathophysiology refers to the disruption of normal bodily functions caused by a disease. Before diabetes sets in, the normal glucose metabolism is a coordinated feedback loop that helps balance glucose production with glucose utilization (primarily by muscle and fat tissue) in the body. This process is aided by insulin, a hormone secreted in the pancreas and released into your bloodstream. A rising glucose level in the blood triggers insulin production. Most of the glucose in your body comes from the food you eat, specifically foods that contain carbohydrates. As shown in Figure 3 on the following page, during the process of digestion, glucose (sugar) enters the bloodstream, and with the help of insulin, is absorbed into the body's cells to be used as energy. This in turn lowers the amount of sugar in the bloodstream. As the blood-sugar level drops, so does the amount of insulin secreted by the pancreas. Both pre-diabetes and diabetes are conditions characterized by impaired glucose tolerance (IGT) and/or impaired fasting glucose (IFG), which indicate a higher than normal glucose level in the blood. As blood-glucose levels continue to rise, the body may develop a state of insulin resistance, which is the body's compensatory mechanism to secrete and release more insulin into the blood. Over time, beta cells (the pancreatic cells that produce insulin) wear out and the pancreas becomes dysfunctional. It is now known that fat tissue does play a major role in glucose regulation, and that excess body fat, especially abdominal fat, is associated with insulin resistance and abnormal glucose metabolism. These conditions, in turn, are associated with a set of abnormal metabolic changes, such as elevated triglycerides, reduced high-density lipoprotein (HDL), and a rise in blood pressure.[20]

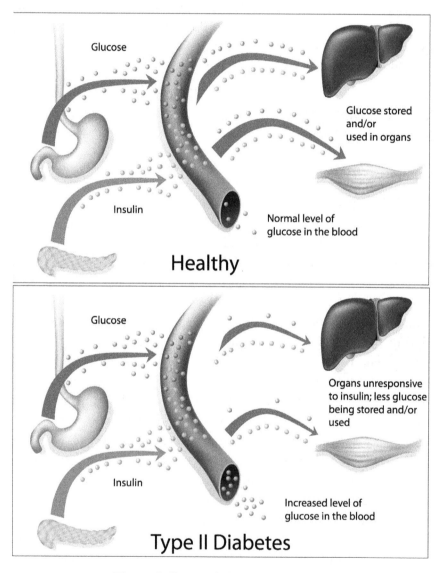

Figure 3. Type-2 diabetes mechanism

DISABILITY AND COMPLICATIONS IN DIABETES

If type-2 diabetes is not controlled or only poorly controlled, the risk for various complications involving multiple organs and systems rises. A vast majority of those with type-2 diabetes eventually die of cardiovascular causes. Other potential life-altering complications include blindness, amputation of lower limbs, kidney failure (nearly 50 percent of Americans receiving kidney dialysis are those with poorly controlled diabetes), and wounds that fail to heal and require frequent interventions.

The most devastating consequences of diabetes are the *macrovascular* (affecting major organs like heart, kidneys and blood vessels) and *microvascular* (affecting smaller organs like the eyes and nervous system) complications it often leads to. Although these complications have many origins and primarily involve the cardiovascular and nervous systems, they may also affect every system in the body.

Cardiovascular Complications

Seventy-five percent of all deaths among people with diabetes are attributed to cardiovascular complications from diabetes. This high propensity for cardiovascular problems among those with diabetes is evidenced by the fact that they have as high a risk for myocardial infarction (MI) as those without diabetes, but with coronary artery disease (CAD). The metabolic abnormalities stemming from diabetes are believed to cause elevated levels of low-density lipoprotein (LDL) cholesterol and triglycerides, higher levels of plasma glucose and insulin, elevated clotting factor (an increased tendency for blood to clot), and high blood pressure, all of which contribute to cardiovascular disease (CVD). As previously stated, the presence of more than one risk factor for any disease exponentially increases the risk for that particular disease due to the synergistic effect of the factors involved. The high incidence of CVD among those with type-2 diabetes has prompted the Joint National Committee on Prevention, Detection, Evaluation, and Treatment of High Blood Pressure, the American Diabetes Association, and the National Cholesterol Education Program to recommend aggressive, multifactorial modification of the risk factors in these individuals. This approach has been found to be highly effective in reducing death, and trauma like amputation from complications of type-2 diabetes.[16] Management of the risk factors involves lifestyle changes to aid in weight loss, smoking cessation, lowering plasma glucose, blood lipids (fats), blood pressure, plus a treatment regimen with antiplatelet agents (e.g., low-dose aspirin), to reduce the risk of blood-vessel blockage.

Hypertension—Complications

Although, technically, hypertension or high blood pressure as a disease state belongs within the cardiovascular group of complications from diabetes, it bears a separate mention because of the severity and the extent of its impact on other vital body organs and systems. A blood pressure reading of 130/80 mm Hg or greater is considered hypertension in individuals with diabetes. Hypertension is twice as common among people with diabetes, compared to people without it, and accounts for 30–70 percent of the complications from diabetes. It also exacerbates other cardiovascular diseases, such as cardiomyopathy (abnormality of the heart that results in its diminished function) and heart failure, renal disease, diabetic retinopathy (disorder of the retina), and stroke. End-stage renal disease is five to six times more likely to develop in those with both hypertension and diabetes, compared to hypertensive people without diabetes. Hypertension quadruples the death rate from diabetes due to its role in the development of associated renal disease and cardiovascular disease.[21]

Diabetic Retinopathy—Complications

While the term retinopathy refers to any disorder of the retina, diabetic retinopathy refers to retinal damage caused by longstanding diabetes that leads to blindness in more than 10,000 people a year. It is the leading cause of blindness in adults under sixty-five years of age, and people with diabetes are 25 times more likely to develop blindness than the general population. More than 60 percent of those with type-2 diabetes develop diabetic retinopathy, and there is evidence that the retinopathy begins to develop long before the formal diagnosis of diabetes is made. In general, the longer the duration of diabetes the more chances there are for the development and increased severity of diabetic retinopathy.[22]

In addition to retinopathy, macular abnormalities, increased incidence of cataracts, and glaucoma also contribute to blindness among people with diabetes. Pregnancy is known to worsen diabetic retinopathy, so when planning to get pregnant, women with diabetes (type-1 or type-2) should undergo a thorough eye examination, then repeat it in the first trimester, and be closely monitored throughout pregnancy for any changes in eye health.

Diabetic Nephropathy—Complications

The term nephropathy refers to kidney disease, and diabetic nephropathy simply means disease of the kidney caused by, or stemming from, diabetes, usually of long duration. The condition is often referred to as a syndrome because it is accompanied by a number of co-existing abnormalities—a high level of albumin in the urine (300 mg or more in a twenty-four hour period), high blood pressure, and a progressive decline in the glomerular filtration rate (GFR), all without any previously known renal disease. Diabetic nephropathy affects about one in five of those with type-2 diabetes, and in the U.S., it is the leading cause of end-stage renal disease (ESRD), accounting for 28,000 new cases each year. ESRD is the number-one reason why people are placed on kidney dialysis, and those with diabetic nephropathy who are on dialysis are known to have a 22-percent higher death rate at one year, and 15-percent higher death rate at five years compared to those without diabetes.[15] Because of the associated high rates of sickness and death, early detection and intervention of diabetic nephropathy are paramount. The American Diabetes Association (ADA) recommends a yearly screening for diabetic nephropathy for those with type-2 diabetes and anyone with type-1 diabetes who has had the disease for at least five years. Lifestyle modifications to lose weight, stop smoking, reduce salt intake, and cut down on alcohol consumption also need to be emphasized for those at high risk of developing diabetic nephropathy.

Diabetic Neuropathy—Complications

This is a condition with signs and symptoms of abnormal function of peripheral nerves in people with diabetes, in the absence of any other causes. Diabetic neuropathy is not a single condition, but multiple disturbances in the peripheral nervous system that all develop as a consequence of *hyperglycemia* (increased blood sugar). The person may or may not experiences symptoms because neuropathy without symptoms is common. Diabetic neuropathies are the most common long-term complications of type-2 diabetes, affecting as many as half the people with diabetes.[15] They may also be found in people with type-1 diabetes, but these are developed over time with the duration of diabetes, and rarely at the time of diagnosis. Diabetic neuropathy is broadly divided into *rapidly reversible hyperglycemic neuropathy,* and *generalized symmetric diabetic polyneuropathy.* The former, as the term implies, may be transient, and is reversible by restoring blood-sugar levels to normal. The generalized variety is characterized by severe sensory symptom, such as pain, a burning sensation, especially in the feet, and an increased sensitivity to sensory stimuli like touch. Improvement occurs slowly with intervention to control the blood-sugar level. Chronic sensorimotor neuropathy, a subtype of diabetic peripheral neuropathy, is the most common form of diabetic neuropathy, and may be present in about 10 percent of those with type-2 diabetes.

Foot Ulceration, Sepsis, and Amputation

Diabetes significantly increases the risk of foot ulceration, and of having a foot ulcer worsens the physical, psychological, and social quality of life among people diagnosed with type-2 diabetes. The prevalence of foot ulcers among those with diabetes is reported to be 4–10 percent, and the lifetime incidence can be as high as 25 percent, while the comparable percentage for the general population ranges from 1.0 to 4.1. There may be several factors at play in developing a foot ulceration, but the most important one is peripheral neuropathy, which is present to some degree in more than 50 percent of those older than sixty years of age who are diagnosed with type-2 diabetes.[23] Other factors that might play a role in causing foot ulceration are excessive plantar pressure related to limited joint mobility, foot deformities, and trauma to the foot, especially when it is repetitive such as that caused by falls, cellulitis, toenail cutting, or the rubbing of ill-fitting shoes.[24]

Obesity and poor vision that are associated with diabetes may also impair effective self-care related to foot ulceration. Evidence to date supports screening anyone with diabetes to identify those at risk for foot ulceration. Certain preventive measures, including patient education, prescription footwear, intensive podiatric care, and evaluation for surgical intervention might benefit those at risk. The most costly and feared consequence of a foot ulcer is limb amputation, which occurs ten to thirty times more often in people with diabetes than in the general population.[25]

Diabetes accounts for 80 percent of non-traumatic amputations, the vast majority of them necessitated by a non-healing foot ulcer. The annual incidence for non-traumatic lower-limb amputations in those with diabetes ranges from 2.1 to 13.7 per 1000 persons. The death rate following amputation in people with diabetes is regarded as being higher than for most malignancies.[26]

ANGEL'S TRANSITION FROM METABOLIC SYNDROME TO DIABETES

Angel is a sixty-eight-year-old man who first came to my office in 1998 for a physical examination. At a height of 5' 2", and weighing 199 pounds, his body mass index (BMI) was 36 (30 and over is considered obese). On the day of the visit, his blood pressure (BP) was 136/90 mm Hg, and his abdominal girth was at 42 inches (over 40" is considered abnormally large for a man). Both his physical examination and his blood tests were otherwise normal.

I explained to Angel that based on his blood pressure and abdominal girth, he met two out of the five criteria for *metabolic syndrome* (a condition marked by a cluster of abnormal metabolic measurements), and told him that it is a disease condition, and a precursor to more serious diseases, such as type-2 diabetes, hypertension, and heart disease. We discussed the importance of his losing weight through diet and exercise in order to prevent any further progression of his existing disease state, as well as forestall the more devastating chronic diseases of diabetes and heart disease.

Over the following six years, Angel kept his weight the same, no gain, no loss, and remained in the obese category. In 2005, his fasting blood glucose (FBG), which up to that point had remained in the normal range, rose to an abnormal level (107 mg/dL) for the first time (normal is 65–99 mg/dL), which put him in the pre-diabetes category. Angel now weighed 202 pounds, still with the same BMI. Since his blood pressure and cholesterol levels were all within normal range, I explained to him that these were in his favor, so he wouldn't get discouraged and stop trying to lose weight. I again emphasized how critical it was for him to lose weight by making some changes in his diet, and adding moderate, regular exercise to his regimen, to improve his overall health as well as to prevent full-blown diabetes and other chronic diseases in the future.

When Angel returned for an office visit three years later in 2008, he had lost three pounds and was back to his old weight of 199 pounds, but his blood pressure (136/72 mm Hg), especially the systolic (upper) number, was higher, and his fasting blood sugar (FBG) of 118 mg/dL was well above normal range. Angel was asked to undergo a two-hour oral glucose tolerance test (OGTT) for a definitive diagnosis of type-2 diabetes, and the results showed that his glucose levels were abnormally high. This confirmed that Angel now had full-blown diabetes as he met the criteria for a diagnosis of type-2 diabetes. To bring his blood-glucose levels under control, he was started on medication and was referred to a nutritionist, and a certified diabetes educator for dietary and lifestyle counseling. In addition, he is being closely monitored for any complications of diabetes that he might develop.

After his diabetes diagnosis, Angel did make some significant lifestyle changes with respect to his diet and exercise, and lost 10 pounds (about 5 percent of his weight) in the first four months. He is currently managing his diabetes well—being diagnosed with diabetes may have been the motivation for Angel to make the needed changes in his diet and lifestyle. Although making the same changes earlier when he was first advised to do so could have prevented his progression to full-blown diabetes, Angel is still reaping the benefits of the lifestyle changes he did make because he is able to halt further progression of his disease, and avert the associated complications.

Angel's case not only illustrates the association between lifestyle and the development of a devastating chronic disease, but it also emphasizes the importance of making the needed lifestyle changes in the early stages of a disease in order to stop its progression to an advanced state with far more serious consequences.

STELLA TOOK CHARGE OF HER HEALTH ONCE SHE WAS DIAGNOSED WITH TYPE-2 DIABETES

Stella, a sixty-two-year-old woman, 5'6" tall, weighing 147 pounds, with a normal body mass index (BMI) of 24, was referred to me in 2008 by her gynecologist, who had noted on more than one occasion, that her blood pressure was elevated. She was not a smoker, drank only moderately—a glass of wine several times a week with her dinner—and, even though she held a sedentary office job, was reported to be fairly physically active off the job. Her family history included two first-degree relatives being treated for hypertension (high blood pressure), one of who also had diabetes. On the day of her visit, Stella's blood pressure was 150/98 mm Hg, which is above the normal level. Her LDL cholesterol and triglycerides were also higher than what is regarded as a normal range for someone with type-2 diabetes. I explained to Stella what her test results meant, and asked her to undergo a two-hour glucose tolerance test (OGTT), which she did promptly. The results of the test also showed an abnormally high (255 mg/dL) blood-glucose level (normal range is 65–140).

Based on the results of her tests, Stella was diagnosed with type-2 diabetes, resulting from insulin deficiency (a latent autoimmune type of diabetes). She was started on medication to treat her diabetes and hyper-cholesterolemia and was referred to a nutritionist and a certified diabetes educator. Stella was also asked to begin a regular exercise program of her liking. Although, she was not overweight, regular exercise would help her maintain her blood glucose at the desired lower levels.

At her follow-up visit four months later, Stella weighed 136 pounds, a loss of 11 pounds or a 7.5-percent reduction from her former weight, and her blood pressure came down from 150/98 mm Hg to 132/84 mm Hg. Both her total cholesterol and LDL cholesterol levels were lower, and within normal range. Stella's hemoglobin A1c was also down to the desired level of 5.8 percent (normal: 4.5%–5.6%), a remarkable overall improvement. As of her last checkup, Stella had both her blood pressure and her diabetes under control through diet, exercise, and medication, and as a result, has not developed any secondary complications from either of her chronic conditions of diabetes or high blood pressure. She achieved these results primarily through making healthier dietary choices that included eating fewer red meats, more leaner meats, and adding more vegetables and fruits, following an exercise regimen of moderate, regular physical activity (all of which helped her lose 7.5 percent of her weight), and, finally, taking prescribed medications without fail.

Stella personifies what can be achieved by combining lifestyle changes and medical intervention to manage a chronic disease. Her success in managing her illness effectively and halting further progression also demonstrates the fact that it takes a concerted effort to make sustained lifestyle changes in order to make a significant difference in the outcome of a chronic disease.

6

Cancer

The word *cancer* refers to not one disease, but to many, all with a common underlying pathology consisting of an uncontrolled growth and spread of abnormal cells, with potentially lethal consequences. To date, more than 200 cancers have been identified. Cancer is the second leading cause of death in the U.S., after cardiovascular diseases, accounting for nearly 1 of every 4 deaths.[1] Available evidence points to the fact that some of the most lethal cancers are attributable to lifestyle choices, such as smoking tobacco, consuming alcohol in excess, poor eating habits that include consumption of excessive amounts of animal products, especially meats cooked at high temperatures and processed meats, physical inactivity, exposure to infectious agents such as human papillomavirus (HPV), hepatitis B virus (HBV), and hepatitis C virus (HCV), as well as exposure to carcinogens in the environment. The environmental carcinogens include chemicals (cigarette smoke is known to contain 3,875 chemicals, some of which are known to cause cancer), prolonged and unprotected exposure to sunlight, and radiation. Also implicated among risk factors for certain types of cancers in women is delayed childbearing (especially of the first child) that deprives women of the protective effect for the reproductive organs of interrupted estrogen production during pregnancy and lactation.

Given what is known about the associated risk factors, it stands to reason that a great many of the cancers could be prevented through behavioral changes that could reduce exposure to the known risk factors and prevent the associated disease conditions through the use of vaccines or antibiotics. All cancers caused by cigarette smoking and heavy use of alcohol could be completely prevented. The World Cancer Research Fund estimates that about 25–33 percent of new cancer cases are related to overweight or obesity, physical inactivity, and poor nutrition, and could be prevented.[2] Many of the more than 2 million skin cancers that are diagnosed annually could be prevented by protecting skin from excessive sun exposure and by avoiding indoor tanning. There are approved screening tests for early detection of some cancers that can result in less extensive treatment and better outcomes. In some cancers, like that of the cervix, colon, and rectum, removal of pre-cancerous growths can prevent a full-blown cancer. Currently, there are standard screening protocols for certain cancers, based on age, gender, and family history. A lack of access to affordable care, especially preventive care, coupled with the long latent phase of cancer prior to symptoms does hinder early detection of cancer. Education to create public awareness of warning signs for certain cancers, and the use of recommended screening, based on age, gender, and risk profiles, can aid in early detection and better outcomes for individuals with those cancers. This is particularly true for colon, skin, and breast cancers. A heightened awareness of changes in the breast or skin through regular self-examination, for example, can result in detection of tumors and lesions at earlier stages, and fewer chances for progression of the disease. Cancer of the lung, breast, colon, prostate, and skin are the most common types of cancers found in the U.S.

HOW PREVALENT IS CANCER?

Cancer is currently the second leading cause of death in the United States, despite a slight decline in recent years, and is expected to surpass heart disease as the leading cause of death in the coming years. The National Cancer Institute estimated that approximately 13.7 million Americans or about 4.4 percent of the population with a history of cancer were alive at the beginning of 2012.[3] The lifetime probability of being diagnosed with an invasive cancer is higher for men (43%) than for women (38%). The reasons for higher susceptibility in men are not yet well understood, but are believed to likely reflect the differences in environmental exposures, gender-specific hormones, and complex interactions between these two. However, for adults aged younger than 50 years, cancer risk is higher for women (5.4%) than for men (3.4%) because of the higher occurrence of breast, genital, and thyroid cancers in young women.

According to a report of its 2010 survey findings by the National Health Interview Survey, eight percent of adults ages eighteen and over in the U.S. had ever been told by a doctor or other health professional that they had some form of cancer.[4] This rate is higher among those age fifty-five or older in terms of ever having been told they had some form of cancer. When the rates are considered by race, non-Hispanic white adults top the list (9 percent) compared to non-Hispanic black adults (5 percent) and Hispanic adults (4 percent). When considering single-race, sex, and ethnicity groups, non-Hispanic white women and men had the highest overall percentages of ever having been told by a doctor or other health professional that they had cancer. The Annual Report to the Nation on the Status of Cancer, 1975–2009, shows that overall cancer death rates continued to decline in the United States among both men and women, all major racial and ethnic groups, and for all of the most common cancer sites, including lung, colon and rectum, breast (female), and prostate.[5] However, the report also pointed out that death rates continued to increase during the latest time period (2000–2009) for cancers of the liver, pancreas, and uterus in women, and melanoma of the skin in men.

The word *cancer* is generally used to refer to malignant tumors that invade surrounding tissues, in contrast to benign tumors that do not. Although, the two may share some overlapping characteristics, benign tumors are rarely life threatening, in contrast to malignant ones that can be, and often are due to their metastatic (spreading) capability. Cancer types are grouped into broader categories based on the affected tissues. For example, any cancer that begins in glandular (secretory) cells responsible for making and releasing substances in the body, such as mucus, digestive juices, or other fluids, is categorized as an *adenocarcinoma.* Most cancers of the breast, pancreas, lung, prostate, and colon fall into this category.

Cancer is caused by both external factors (tobacco, infectious organisms, chemicals, and radiation) and internal factors (inherited mutations, hormones, immune conditions, and mutations that occur from metabolism). These factors may all act together or in sequence to initiate or promote the development of cancer—ten or more years often pass between exposure to external factors and a detectable cancer due to the long latency period that's characteristic of the disease. The probability an individual will develop or die from cancer (of any kind) over the course of a lifetime is referred to as the *lifetime risk,* and this estimate is based on the incidence and mortality data for all invasive cancers for men and women. In the United States, the National Cancer Institute determined that men have slightly less than a 1 in 2 lifetime risk of developing cancer, and a 1 in 4 risk of dying from cancer, while the corresponding risks for women are 1 in 3, and 1 in 5, respectively.[6] It is, however, important to note that these estimates are based on the average experience of the general population and may over- or underestimate individual risk because of differences in exposure (e.g. smoking), and/or genetic susceptibility.

SURVIVING CANCER

The survival rate for all cancers has been steadily improving, reflecting both progress in diagnosing certain cancers at an earlier stage, and improvements in treatment of others. Relative survival compares survival among cancer patients to that of people of the same age, race, and sex who are not diagnosed with cancer. Although the five-year relative survival rate for all cancers as a group continues to improve, the rates vary greatly by type of cancer and disease stage when diagnosed. The rate represents the percentage of people with cancer who are alive after some designated time period (usually five years, but can be less or more depending on the type of cancer) relative to those without cancer. It does not distinguish between those who have been cured, are still in treatment, or those for whom the disease has relapsed. The survival rate also does not capture deaths that occur beyond the designated time period (for example, five years) after diagnosis. The relative survival rate is useful, however, to monitor progress in the early detection and treatment of cancer, as early detection and intervention do improve survival rates even in the deadliest forms of cancer, such as lung cancer.

LUNG CANCER

According to a 2014 report released by the American Cancer Society, lung cancer is the leading cause of cancer death in the United States for both men and women.[7] Worldwide, lung cancer is the leading cause of cancer death in men, and the second leading cause of cancer death in women.[8] Overall, the chance that a man will develop lung cancer in his lifetime is about 1 in 13; for a woman, the risk is about 1 in 16. Lung cancer is more commonly found in older persons, the average age at the time of diagnosis being around seventy years, and fewer than two percent of all cases are found in people younger than forty-five. Over the past two decades, the lung-cancer rate has been dropping among men and has just recently begun to drop in women. Many in public health and epidemiology attribute this to a drop in smoking rates.

The type of lung cancer is identified by the size of affected cell and/ or the location of tumor within the lung.

- **Small-cell lung cancer (SCLC).** Named for the size of the cancer cells when seen under a microscope, this is a less common type found in only about 10–15 percent of lung cancers. This cancer is also known as oat cell cancer, oat cell carcinoma, and small cell undifferentiated carcinoma. It is predominantly found in smokers, and is very rare among those who have never smoked.

- **Non-small-cell lung cancer (NSCLC).** This is the most common type of lung cancer, found in about 85–90 percent of lung cancers.[9] It often starts in the bronchi near the center of the lung and tends to spread widely through the body of the lung fairly early in the course of the disease. There are three main subtypes of NSCLC, plus a few less common ones. These cancer cells differ in size, shape, and chemical make-up, but their treatment and prognosis for those affected are often very similar.

- **Squamous cell carcinoma.** Found in about 25–30 percent of all lung cancers, this lung cancer is most often linked to a history of smoking. The cancer starts in the cells that line the inside of the airways in the lungs and is likely to be found in the middle of the lungs, near a bronchus.

  - **Adenocarcinoma.** Found in about 40 percent of lung cancers, this cancer starts in cells that normally secrete such substances as mucus. This type is more commonly seen in non-smokers, but is also found in current or former smokers. It is more common in women than in men, and is more likely to occur at a younger age than other types of lung cancer. Adenocarcinoma is usually found in outer parts of the lung, and tends to grow slower than other types of lung cancer, and is more likely to be detected before it has spread outside of the lung. It is known to have a better prognosis than other types of lung cancer.

- **Large cell (undifferentiated) carcinoma.** This subtype of cancer accounts for about 10–15 percent of lung cancers. It can appear in any part of the lung, and tends to grow and spread quickly, which can make it harder to treat, and thus has a poor prognosis.

Origin and Spread of Lung Cancer

Lung cancers are known to start as areas of pre-cancerous changes in the lung. The changes in the genes (DNA) inside the lung cells may cause the cells to grow rapidly, indicative of an abnormal cell change. These cells may look abnormal if seen under a microscope, but they have not formed into a mass or tumor that can be seen on an x-ray. At this stage, the person does not experience any symptoms. Over time, the abnormal cells may undergo other gene changes that cause them to progress to full-blown cancer. As the cancer develops, new blood vessels are formed in the area to nourish and grow the cancer cells, which, over time, form into a tumor large enough to be seen on imaging tests, such as x-rays and scans. Some of the cancer cells may break away from the original tumor at some point, and spread (metastasize) to other parts of the body. Lung cancer is more often than not a life-threatening disease, more so than the other cancers, because it tends to spread before it can be detected on an imaging test like a chest x-ray.

The term *lymph node* is often used in conjunction with a diagnosis of cancer. The lymphatic system is one of the ways in which cancers spread from their primary site of origin to other parts of the body. The lymphatic system consists of lymph nodes (small, bean-shaped collections of immune-system cells that fight infections), and is connected by lymphatic vessels that are similar to small veins, but carry a clear fluid called *lymph* away from the lungs. Lymph contains excess fluid and waste products from body tissues in addition to the immune-system cells. Lung-cancer cells can enter lymphatic vessels and begin to grow in lymph nodes around the bronchi and in the mediastinum (the area between the lungs). Once these cells have reached the lymph nodes, they are more likely to have spread to other organs of the body as well. The staging (extent) of the cancer and any decisions about treatment are based in part on whether or not the cancer has spread to the nearby lymph nodes in the mediastinum.

KNOWN RISK FACTORS FOR LUNG CANCER

Smoking Tobacco

More than half a century ago, epidemiologists recognized smoking as a major risk factor for lung cancer. In 1964, the Surgeon General's Report, *Smoking and Health,* was released. It was the culmination of an in-depth exploration of the effects of smoking on health by a committee of experts from a wide range of biomedical fields that used data from several major epidemiological studies. Included among these were three large, prospective studies, one of which used British doctors as participants.

There are two ways to gather data from participants in a study. The retrospective method of gathering data starts with two groups of people, one with the disease and the other without the disease, and gathers the participants' smoking history going back in time. This method of study relies on participants' recall of their smoking habits, and is considered flawed because of the tendency of people *with* lung cancer to overestimate, and for those *without* the disease to under-estimate the amount they smoked. The prospective method of study begins with two groups of healthy (disease-free) participants, one of smokers and the other nonsmokers, and follows them into the future, ensuring that, other than the smoking habit, the two groups are comparable in all relevant factors, such as age, sex, race, and socioeconomic status. The disease and death rates between the two groups are compared as they unfold over time. In all three prospective studies done for the report, the researchers found that the death rates from lung cancer were far higher among smokers than nonsmokers. The ratio of deaths for heavy smokers relative to non-smokers was 20 to 1 in two of the studies, and 40 to 1 in the third, a finding that helped confirm and quantify the excess risk from smoking in lung-cancer deaths. Examining the relationship between the amount of smoking and lung cancer, researchers also noted that the death rates were higher for each successive increment of the amount smoked. These and similar studies of the association between smoking and lung cancer attested to the strength of this association. The incremental positive link between the two helped establish the *dose-response* (more smoking leads to more deaths) nature of the association between smoking and lung cancer deaths.

Since these early studies were published, hundreds more have been done to further explore this association, necessitated, in part, by the tobacco industry's persistent efforts to refute the findings of earlier studies pointing out the strong positive association between cigarette smoking and lung cancer. The later studies not only confirmed the earlier findings, but also added to them by demonstrating that both the amount and duration (in years) of smoking had the effect of increasing the risk for developing lung cancer, and dying from it, in effect establishing beyond doubt that smoking carries with it an excessive risk for lung cancer. The magnitude of the excess lung-cancer risk among cigarette smokers relative to non-smokers makes a persuasive case for supporting the theory of a causal relationship between lung cancer and cigarette smoking.

Tobacco smoked via pipes and cigars does not appear to carry the same degree of increased risk for lung cancer, but is associated with an increased risk of cancer of the *buccal* (cheek) cavity and larynx (vocal cord). Based on this evidence, researchers have concluded that the increased lung-cancer risk is associated with increased cigarette smoking, but not with increased consumption of tobacco in other forms. Nevertheless, it bears repeating that tobacco remains the leading preventable cause of disease, disability, and death in the U.S. Establishing the indisputable link between cigarette smoking and lung cancer is one of the most significant contributions to public health made by epidemiology in the past 60 years.

THE MECHANISM BY WHICH SMOKING TOBACCO MAY LEAD TO LUNG CANCER

It is estimated that tobacco smoke contains at least 3875 different chemicals, and at least fifty-five of these are recognized as carcinogens (substances capable of causing or increasing chances of developing cancer in humans or animals). Based on studies of laboratory animals, the available data all points to the probable involvement of twenty substances in the development of lung cancer due to their demonstrated lung carcinogenicity.[10] Long-term exposure to these carcinogens by smokers is known to cause multiple genetic changes at the cellular level. It is, therefore, plausible that, over time, the DNA damage produced by carcinogens in the tobacco smoke causes the multiple genetic changes that are associated with lung cancer. In quantitative terms, while the amount of carcinogen delivered from a single cigarette is extremely small, the cumulative damage caused by years of smoking is substantial. There are other explanations in the literature about the mechanisms by which smoking induces lung cancer, but the one stated above is most consistent with the existing understanding of the underlying pathology in lung cancer.

Particle Pollution

Particle pollution, a mix of very tiny solid and liquid particles in the air everyone breathes, has been recognized as one of the risk factors for lung cancer because concentrations of measured particle matter in recent decades have been linked to small but measurable increases in deaths from lung cancer. Studies have conclusively shown that breathing high levels of particle pollution year-round can be deadly as it causes significant damage to the small airways of lungs. This, in turn, has been linked with an increased risk of dying from lung cancer, among other serious cardiopulmonary illnesses in both children and adults.[11] Particles in the air are of different sizes, some as small as one-tenth the diameter of a strand of hair, and others are even smaller, and can only be seen with an electron microscope. While you can't see the individual particles, you can see the haze that forms in the atmosphere when millions of particles blur the spread of sunlight. The particle size makes a difference in how particle pollution affects you. Your natural defenses help you cough or sneeze larger particles out of your body, but those defenses don't work for keeping out smaller, microscopic particles. No matter what size they are, particles get trapped in the lungs, and the smallest are so minute that they can pass through the lungs into the bloodstream.

Particle pollution is produced through mechanical and chemical processes. Mechanical processes primarily create coarse particles from dust storms, construction and demolition, mining operations, road wear from traffic, agriculture, pollen, mold, and plant and animal debris. By contrast, chemical processes in the atmosphere create most of the fine and ultrafine particles, primarily from combustion sources that burn fuels and emit gases. Burning fossil fuels in factories, power plants, steel mills, smelters, diesel- and gasoline-powered motor vehicles (despite the prevailing emission standards) and equipment generate a large percentage of the raw materials for fine particles. Burning wood in residential fireplaces and wood stoves, or burning agricultural fields and forests also contribute to particle pollution.

Particles are composed of many different compounds, and vary between different regions in the United States, and at different times of the year. For example, on average, the Midwest, Southeast, and Northeast states have more sulfate particles than the West, primarily due to the high levels of sulfur dioxide emitted by large, coal-fired power plants, whereas nitrate particles from motor-vehicle exhaust dominate the unhealthful particle mix in Southern California, the Northwest, and the North Central U.S. Studies have shown that breathing air polluted with particles can trigger illness, hospitalization, and premature death, and that reducing air pollution improves the health and quality of life.[12] Based on the available evidence, the Environmental Protection Agency (EPA) also came to a similar conclusion that particle pollution causes multiple serious threats to health.[13]

Radon Gas

Exposure to residential radon gas is a major source of ionizing radiation in most countries. Underground miners are also exposed to radon and its byproducts. A group of researchers analyzed data from thirteen different European studies on the association between exposure to radon gas and an increase in risk for lung cancer.[14] Their findings pointed to an average 8.4 percent increase in risk for lung cancer (ranging from 3–15.8 percent) due to radon-gas exposure. The associated rise in risk with radon exposure was significantly higher among smokers than nonsmokers, a reflection of the synergistic effect of the two agents involved. Evidence from the pooled European studies led the researchers to conclude that, in the absence of other causes, the risk for lung cancer from exposure to radon gas at the usual concentrations is about twenty-five times greater among cigarette smokers than among lifelong non-smokers, a finding that was corroborated by studies done in the U.S. and Canada. These studies also revealed an incremental increase in lung cancer connected to an incremental increase in exposure to radon gas, indicative of a dose-response relationship between the two.

Low-Dose Radiation

Estimates of lung-cancer risk after exposure to radiation are based on studies of people exposed to it at high rates, such as the atomic-bomb survivors. However, research in radiobiology and animal experiments suggests that risks from exposure to radiation at low to moderate rates, such as that delivered by medical diagnostic procedures like X-rays, may be overestimated. From 1950 to 1987, a study of low-dose radiation and lung-cancer mortality was done on a large cohort (64,172) of Canadian tuberculosis patients. Thirty-nine percent were exposed to multiple chest fluoroscopies and received moderate doses of radiation. Data on the deaths from lung cancer gathered on these test subjects were compared directly to estimates derived from 75,991 atomic bomb survivors. Based on 1,178 lung-cancer deaths among people with tuberculosis, the researchers concluded there was no evidence that the diagnostic procedures were responsible for any excess radiation risk. In other words, the people in this study were not at any increased risk of dying from lung cancer than the general population.[15] This implies that the risk of lung cancer from exposure to radiation at the current low-to-medium dose rates used in medical procedures is significantly lower than the high-dose-rate exposures such as those emitted by atomic bombs, and did not pose a threat to health. The evidence from studies done on nuclear-industry workers in many countries to determine the risk for cancer deaths from exposure to low-level, external, predominantly γ radiation (Gamma rays or Gamma radiation) is also consistent with findings from this large study.[16] The analyses of data from studies with nuclear workers covered a total of 2,124,526 person-years (PY) at risk and 15,825 deaths, 3,976 of which were due to cancer. Based on these findings, researchers concluded that there is no evidence of an association between Gamma radiation dose and deaths from all causes or from cancers of any type. These estimates are the most comprehensive and precise direct estimates obtained to date of cancer risk associated with exposures to long-term, low-dose ionizing radiation. The combination of the data from studies done in multiple countries and settings, yielding consistent results, increases the level of confidence that can be placed in the findings.

Asbestos

Exposure to asbestos has been linked with mesothelioma, chronic obstructive pulmonary disease (COPD), and others, but the association between the risk for lung cancer and asbestos has not been clearly established to-date. There are three main types of asbestos— *crocidolite, amosite,* and *chrysotile,* commonly known as the blue, brown, and white asbestos respectively. Exposure to the *crocidolite* or *amosite* types of asbestos has been associated with a small but measurable risk in lung cancer, ranging between 1–5 percent, but the effect of exposure to *chrysotile* on lung cancer risk is less clear, with inconsistent patterns observed. Statistically, after adjustment for smoking, elevated risks for lung cancer from asbestos were seen among those who worked in industries dealing with metal production and processing, transportation, and freight handling, vehicle-engine building and installation, and rubber and plastics production. The relative risk of lung cancer due to asbestos exposure has been found to be the same for smokers and non-smokers, suggesting the absence of a synergy effect between smoking and asbestos with respect to lung cancer.

THE NATURAL HISTORY OF LUNG CANCER

Despite the identification of several factors that increase the risk for lung cancer decades ago, actually delineating the stages in the natural history of lung cancer has been challenging and was considered a moot point because, by the time the lung cancer is detected, it is often fatal, even at stage I. Studies of lung-cancer screening have not yet been able to establish that, for a period before a lung cancer becomes advanced and fatal, it is localized and treatable. Instead, these studies suggest that the early-stage lung cancers identified by screening are not precursors of the advanced and more fatal disease.

LUNG CANCER CLAIMED TWO LIVES
IN ONE FAMILY—BOTH WERE SMOKERS

Sara, a 68-year-old woman, was my patient for nearly 20 years. In early 2015, she came to see me for a cough and wheezing that she had had for about two weeks. She had no other signs or symptoms suggestive of an infection. Sara did not have asthama or history of any other respiratory problems. She was being treated for high blood pressure at the time. I ordered a chest x-ray for Sara, which was done on the same day she came to see me. The x-ray showed an opaque area in Sara's left lung, suggestive of a possible pneumonia or a mass in her lung. A computer tomography (CT Scan), also done on the same day, confirmed the presence of a mass. I immediately referred Sara to a pulmonologist who performed a bronchoscopy on her, and did a biopsy of the tissue from the suspicious mass. The results of the biopsy led to a diagnosis of Adenocarcinoma (a type of lung cancer). In order to determine the extent of the spread of her cancer, Sara had MRI (magnetic resonance imaging) of her brain, which showed the presence of spread, and a subsequent PET scan revealed that the cancer has spread widely in her body, including her liver and bones. Sara received chemotherapy from a medical oncologist, but her cancer did not respond well to the treatment. Sara died 11 months later at her home.

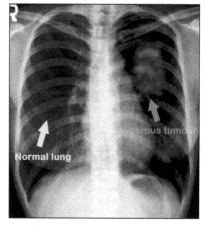

Figure 4. X-Ray of Lung Cancer in Woman

Sara had been a former smoker, but had not smoked in the 20 years prior to her diagnosis of lung cancer. However, her husband William had been a smoker for most of his life, was diagnosed with metastatic lung cancer, and died from it five years earlier. So, Sara was exposed to second-hand smoke, even after she quit smoking herself. In this case, tobacco smoke claimed tragically not one, but two lives from the same family.

BREAST CANCER

Breast cancer in the United States is the most common cancer in women, no matter what race or ethnicity, and is the second most common cause of death from cancer among women, the most common being lung cancer. It is now estimated that one in eight women will develop invasive breast cancer over the course of her life. This lifetime risk is based on current incidence rates, and translates to 12.4 percent of the women born in the United States today developing breast cancer at some time during their lives.[17] This estimate is based on breast cancer statistics for the years 2007 through 2009 and, to date, no further revisions have been made on the risk estimate. This means that, if the current incidence rate stays the same, a female child born today has about a one in eight chance of being diagnosed with breast cancer at some time during her life; this also means the chance that she will *never* have breast cancer is 87.6 percent, or about seven in eight. In the 1970s, the lifetime risk for a woman being diagnosed with breast cancer in the United States was just under one in ten, and since then the risk has risen incrementally to the current level. Men do get breast cancer, but male breast cancer is not common, accounting for less than two percent of all breast-cancer cases. In men, breast cancer can happen at any age, but is most common in men who are between sixty and seventy years of age.

The breast is made up of three main parts—glands, ducts, and connective tissue. The glands secrete milk for lactation, the ducts carry the milk to the nipple, and the connective tissue (consisting of fibrous and fatty tissue) connects and holds all the breast parts together. The way breasts look and feel can be affected by the menstrual period, having had children, losing or gaining weight, taking certain medications, and aging.

Lumps in the Breast that are not Cancerous

Many conditions can cause lumps in the breast, including cancer, but most breast lumps are caused by other medical conditions. The two most common causes of breast lumps are fibrocystic breast condition, and cysts. The fibrocystic condition causes noncancerous changes in the breasts that can make them lumpy, tender, and sore. Cysts are small fluid-filled sacs that can develop in the breast.

Types of Breast Cancer

Breast cancer can begin in different parts of the breast, such as the ducts or the lobes. The type of breast cancer depends on which breast cells turn cancerous. The following are the most common.

- **Ductal carcinoma.** This is the most common kind of breast cancer, and it begins in the cells that line the ducts in the breast.

- **Ductal carcinoma in situ (DCIS).** In this type, the abnormal cancer cells are only in the lining of the milk ducts and have not spread to other tissues in the breast.

- **Invasive ductal carcinoma.** The abnormal cancer cells in this type break through the ducts and spread to other parts of the breast tissue. Invasive cancer cells can also spread to other parts of the body.

- **Lobular carcinoma.** In this kind of breast cancer, the cancer cells begin in the lobes, or lobules, of the breast, which are the glands that produce milk.

- **Lobular carcinoma in situ (LCIS).** The cancer cells are found only in the breast lobules. Lobular carcinoma in situ, or LCIS, does not spread to other tissues.

- **Invasive lobular carcinoma.** Cancer cells spread from the lobules to the nearby breast tissues. These invasive cancer cells can also spread to other parts of the body.

There are also several other less common types of breast cancer, such as Paget's disease or inflammatory breast cancer.

Risk Factors for Breast Cancer

The causes of breast cancer are still poorly understood with known breast-cancer risk factors explaining only a small proportion of cases. However, research on breast cancer over the past several decades has identified multiple factors associated with an increased risk for developing the disease. These risk factors fall into four categories— demographic (age and gender primarily, but country of origin, and socioeconomic status also play a role), hormonal, familial or genetic, and lifestyle related.

- **Age and gender.** Female age and gender are both major non-modifiable risk factors for breast cancer. The highest rate of breast-cancer incidence is reported in women between fifty and seventy years of age. The rate is reported to be increasing, particularly among women ages fifty to sixty-four, and is possibly attributable to better detection by mammography screening in this age group. Breast cancer accounts for about a fifth of all deaths in women between the ages of forty and fifty years.[18] Aging alone poses the greatest risk for breast cancer among women. A 57 percent increase in the cumulative risk of breast cancer by age seventy has been documented. As mentioned earlier, breast cancer can and does occur in men, but the incidence is extremely low, accounting for less than 2 percent of all diagnosed breast cancer cases.

- **Hormonal and reproductive factors.** Increased lifetime exposure to estrogen is linked to an increased risk of breast cancer. Because of this, women who were younger than twelve years of age when they had their first menstrual period, as well as women who started menopause after the age of forty-five, are considered at increased risk for breast cancer. Also included in this category of higher risk for breast cancer are women who gave birth to their first child after the age of thirty, those who have never given birth, and those who never breastfed. Conversely, later onset of menstruation (after age twelve), early childbearing (first full-term pregnancy before twenty years of age), multiple pregnancies (five or more full-term), and early menopause (before forty-five years of age) are associated with a reduced risk of breast cancer due to reduced lifetime exposure to the estrogen hormone.

• **Oral Contraceptives.** The subject of whether or not the use of oral contraceptives increases the risk of breast cancer later in life has been thoroughly investigated in multiple population-based, case-control studies of former and current users of oral contraceptives. Among women from thirty-five to sixty-four years of age, current or former oral-contraceptive use was not associated with a significantly increased risk of breast cancer. The relative risk also did not increase consistently with longer periods of use or with higher doses of estrogen, or the initiation of oral-contraceptive use at a younger age.[19] The use of oral contraceptives by women with a family history of breast cancer was also not found to be associated with an increased risk of breast cancer attributable to oral contraceptive use in these women.[20] The long-term use of hormone replacement therapy is, however, associated with a modest increase in the risk for breast cancer. The combination therapy with both estrogen and progesterone (used by women who have their uterus intact) is associated with a greater increase in risk than estrogen-alone therapy (used by women who had their uterus removed by surgery).[21]

• **Exposure to radiation.** Radiation, especially to the chest wall, has been found to increase a woman's risk for breast cancer, in particular if she was exposed to it between the ages of ten and thirty years of age.[22]

• **Familial factor.** A family history of breast cancer in one or more first-degree relatives (mother, father, sister, brother, daughter, or son) is associated with increased risk of breast cancer, especially if one of these relatives was diagnosed with breast cancer prior to age fifty. A history of ovarian cancer, or both breast and ovarian cancer in a first-degree relative or in two second-degree relatives (grandmother, granddaughter, aunt, or niece) also increases a woman's risk of developing breast cancer. A history of benign (non-cancerous) breast disease, abnormal findings on a previous breast biopsy, and treatment with radiation to the breast or chest are all associated with an increased risk of breast cancer. Dense breast tissue, as detected by mammography, is also associated with increased risk for breast cancer, one theory behind this being that dense breast tissue makes it more difficult to visualize abnormalities. In some states in the U.S. (e.g. California), laws have been introduced to not only inform the women of this mammography finding, but also to advise them to have a follow-up breast ultrasound.

- **Genetic factors.** There are over twenty genes identified as contributing to inherited breast cancers. Of these, the two most recognized mutations that are known to contribute 60 percent of inherited breast cancers are BRCA1 (breast cancer gene 1) and BRCA2 (breast cancer gene 2). The BRCA genes are most prevalent in, but not limited to, people of Ashkenazi Jewish descent. The lifetime risk of breast cancer among Ashkenazi Jewish women carrying the gene mutation has been reported to be as high as 82 percent in some studies, and the risk appears to be increasing with time—by age fifty, the risk among carriers of the BRCA gene born before 1940 was estimated to be 24 percent, but among those born after 1940 the estimate was elevated to 67 percent. During the same time period, the lifetime risks of ovarian cancer were 54 percent for BRCA1 and 23 percent for BRCA2 mutation carriers.[23] BRCA gene testing can help determine the breast-cancer risk status, especially if a woman is known to be at high risk because of a strong family history of breast cancer. The US Preventive Services Task Force (USPSTF) supports genetic testing in such women. Overall, however, genetic mutations are believed to account for only 3–5 percent of diagnosed breast cancers.[24]

- **Lifestyle factors.** Diet has been closely studied for its association with breast-cancer risk, but to date there has not been any consistent positive or negative association with food, including meats, fruits, and vegetables, the phytoestrogens commonly found in soy products, or coffee, tea and other beverages containing caffeine. However, among women, alcohol consumption beyond one drink per day is associated with a significant and incremental rise in the risk for breast cancer. According to some estimates, beyond one drink a day, the incremental rise in risk is as much as 7 percent per drink.[25] Unlike lung cancer, smoking has shown no appreciable impact on the risk for breast cancer.

- **Overweight and obesity.** Both are associated with an increased risk for breast cancer, particularly in postmenopausal women. The association is incremental as the risk increases with increasing body mass index (BMI). The relative risk (risk compared to women of normal weight) in obese postmenopausal women (BMI greater than thirty) is reported to be 1.59 times, and in those who are forty-four pounds (twenty kg) or more over normal weight, the risk to be twice that of normal-weight women. The association of overweight and obesity with increased cancer risk has been explained, at least in part, by alterations in the metabolism of endogenous hormones, which can lead to a distortion of the normal balance between cell proliferation, differentiation, and the life cycle of cells.[26]

- **Lack of regular exercise.** Although there is no evidence to date that habitual physical inactivity increases the risk for breast cancer, regular exercise, even of moderate intensity has been shown to reduce relative risk for breast cancer by as much as 30 percent in premenopausal women, and from 11–22 percent in postmenopausal women, depending on the intensity of the activity, and the leanness of the person. Regular exercise has been shown to have greater beneficial effect on lean women in reducing the relative risk for breast cancer.

Among the long list of factors described above, some, such as the age, female gender, a family history of breast cancer, and being a carrier of the BRCA1 and BRCA2 genes are not modifiable. But such other factors as hormone therapy, alcohol consumption, excess body weight, and physical activity are modifiable. The concerted efforts of many private, voluntary, and public entities to create awareness about the known risk factors for breast cancer, and the importance of being screened for early detection of breast cancer are having some success, as is demonstrated by the steadily improving breast-cancer survival rates.

THE NATURAL HISTORY OF BREAST CANCER

The susceptibility to breast cancer begins with exposure to one or more of the risk factors described above. Development of the disease involves a confluence of factors, generally in play over an extended period of time.

The disease process encompasses progressive changes from normal breast tissue to carcinoma in situ (cancer has not yet begun to spread), then ultimately to invasive carcinoma (cancer has spread to other organs and tissues), as shown in the figure below. Some differences in the natural history of different types of breast cancer do exist. The earliest recognizable symptom of breast cancer is an easily noticeable mass in the breast that is detected on self-examination or during clinical breast examination by a healthcare provider. The mass is generally painless and can vary from the size of a pea to the size of a golf ball (it's unusual to go undetected until it reaches this size, but that has been reported). A metastasis (spread) to the axillary (armpit) lymph nodes is determined by the size of the primary tumor, which is a reflection of the quantity of cancer cells in the tumor (see Figure 5).

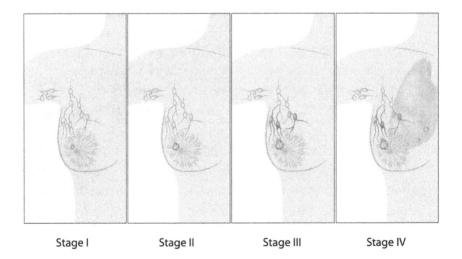

| Stage I | Stage II | Stage III | Stage IV |

Figure 5. Stages in Breast Cancer

Any obvious suspicious mass needs to be investigated further by radiological (mammogram, scanning) or histological (biopsy) diagnostic methods for a definitive diagnosis. The tumor size, grade, involvement of axillary lymph nodes, and other indications of the cancer spreading to other organs and areas of the body determine the course of treatment and the prognosis for survival. As with other chronic diseases, early detection of breast cancer is key to a better prognosis and longer survival.

THE CONSEQUENCES OF IGNORING PREVENTIVE HEALTH ADVICE

Karen, a sixty-nine-year-old woman, came in for a routine physical examination. At a height of 5' 4", she weighed 125 pounds with a normal body mass index (BMI) of 21, and had normal blood pressure on the day of the visit. All findings of her physical examination, including the clinical breast exam, were also normal. Her medical history revealed a partial bowel resection for a pre-malignant tumor several years before. She also reported that she was currently being treated for hypertension (high blood pressure) and low bone density (osteopenia). Karen had smoked for thirty-six years before she quit in her early sixties. She had one child at age thirty-one and became menopausal at age fifty-two. There was a strong family history of cardiovascular disease, but not cancer. Since Karen had not had a mammogram in over five years, she was asked to schedule one, and was also given a laboratory requisition for blood tests, but she did not follow through with either of these.

About eight months later, Karen noticed a change in the texture of her skin around the nipple of her right breast, and came to the office to consult me about it. After examining the area, I confirmed that there was indeed a difference in the texture of the skin in the area she pointed out, and that it warranted a diagnostic mammogram immediately, and sent her to the radiologist the same day to have a mammogram. The radiologist, who saw the results, followed the mammogram with a more detailed imaging that showed a sub-areolar (underneath the nipple) irregular mass measuring one centimeter, as well as an abnormal looking lymph node in the right axilla (armpit). A needle biopsy revealed Karen had invasive ductal carcinoma (cancer) of her right breast, and a positive axillary lymph node indicating a metastasis (spread to other tissues). As the cancer had spread to her lymph node, Karen underwent a whole-body scan, and CT scans to detect any spread beyond that, but the cancer had not spread to her bone, chest, abdomen, or pelvis. Karen underwent a central breast lumpectomy followed by whole breast radiation therapy and a course of chemotherapy. She is now taking daily hormonal therapy and is tolerating it well to date.

The takeaway from Karen's case is that, despite her past medical history involving surgery for a pre-malignant tumor (pre-cancerous) in a different part of her body, she neglected to follow through with a clinician's recommendation to have a mammogram. It was eight months later, taking her cue from visible changes in her breast, that she sought medical attention. By that time, her cancer had spread to an adjacent lymph node. While it is impossible to determine what difference the eight months may have made in the progression of her cancer, it's clear that Karen did not do herself any favors by waiting. As has been mentioned in the book, in several contexts, poor lifestyle choices are often seen in clusters. In Karen's case her thirty-six-year smoking history and her failure to utilize preventive health services, even when prompted, are the two choices she made, both modifiable risks for cancer, that did not serve her well.

JULIA MADE GOOD LIFESTYLE CHOICES, BUT STILL HAD CANCER BECAUSE OF TWO NON-MODIFIABLE RISK FACTORS SHE FACED.

Julia is a sixty-seven-year-old woman I saw in my office for a routine physical examination. She had no particular complaints, but had a past medical history of hypertension (abnormally high blood pressure) for which she was taking medication. She also was taking calcium, and vitamin D for previously diagnosed osteopenia (low bone density). Julia had bilateral breast augmentation several years before. Her gyneco-logical history included having her first child at the age of twenty-two and experiencing menopause at the age of fifty-nine. Her family history revealed that her maternal grandmother had had breast cancer. Julia did not smoke, and drank alcohol only on occasion. At a height of 5' 5", she weighed 145 pounds, with a normal body mass index (BMI) of 24. The findings of her entire physical examination, including a clinical breast exam and vital signs, were normal. Julia was asked to have a mammogram and a blood test done for screening and assessment, which she promptly complied with. After receiving and reviewing the results of her tests, I noted that her blood test results were normal, but her mammogram results revealed that she had dense breasts and a suspi-cious mass in the upper outer quadrant of her left breast. This caused the radiologist to recommended additional breast imaging. Subsequent additional imaging and a breast biopsy showed that Julia had invasive ductal carcinoma (cancer) of the left breast. Shortly thereafter, she was scheduled for a left breast lumpectomy, to be later followed by a partial brachytherapy (breast radiation therapy) and hormonal therapy. Her axil-lary lymph-node biopsy was negative for cancer spread, so Julia did not require chemotherapy. In order to prevent a recurrence of the cancer in the same breast or development of a new cancer in the second breast, she will continue hormonal therapy for at least five years.

Julia's exposure to two known risk factors—a family history of breast cancer in a second-degree relative (a grandmother), and having dense breasts (both non-modifiable risk factors)—increased her chances of developing breast cancer and delaying its detection. Dense breasts, though not known to directly contribute to the development of cancer, make visualization of breast tissue on imaging difficult, making early detection of tumor growth more challenging. Dense breasts thus indi-rectly contribute to a delayed diagnosis, and a worse prognosis. Newer breast-imaging techniques, however, make it possible to overcome this hurdle and make dense breast tissue less of a factor in the diagnosis of breast cancer.

COLORECTAL CANCER

Colorectal cancer is the third most commonly diagnosed cancer in both men and women, and is the third leading cause of cancer death in the U.S.[27] This cancer most often develops in the colon or the rectum, and only infrequently in the small intestine. The disease often begins as non-cancerous growths called polyps. Though most polyps will not become cancerous, their detection through appropriate screening procedures, followed by their removal can prevent a potential colon cancer from developing. In the U.S., colorectal cancer rates vary widely by geographic area. This is attributed to regional variations in exposure to risk factors, legislative policies, and socioeconomic factors that determine access to, and utilization of screening, and treatment facilities and services. Age-adjusted rates of colorectal cancer among men are highest in Alaskan natives, followed by Japanese Americans, and then African-Americans. Among women, the rate is highest for Alaskan native women, followed by African-American women, and then white women. However, death rates for colorectal cancer are substantially higher among African American men, followed by Alaskan natives, and then people of Hawaiian Islands. There has been significant progress in reducing colorectal cancer incidence and death rates in most U.S. population groups, primarily through prevention and early detection by screening. In the past decade, the rapid decline in rates has also been attributed to the detection and removal of pre-cancerous polyps. Since 1998, rates have been declining by 3.0 percent a year in men and 2.3 percent a year in women.[28] Further progress can be made by increasing wider access to colorectal cancer screening tests. Only a little over half of the people age fifty or older, for whom screening is highly recommended, report having had colorectal cancer screening.[29]

Major Risk Factors for Colorectal Cancer

There are many known factors associated with either the increased or decreased risk of developing colorectal cancer. Some factors linked to increased risk are modifiable, while others are non-modifiable. The

latter include a personal history of polyps, or a family history of colorectal cancer or polyps, and a personal history of chronic inflammatory
bowel disease. The American Cancer Society and other organizations
recommend that people at increased risk for colorectal cancer because
of these factors begin screening at an earlier age than is recommended
for individuals with average-risk (*see* chapter 9). In epidemiologic
studies, modifiable risk factors associated with an increased risk of
colorectal cancer are shown to include physical inactivity, obesity, a
high consumption of red or processed meats, smoking, and moder-
ate-to-heavy alcohol consumption. A recent study found that about
one-quarter of colorectal cancer cases could be avoided by following a
healthy lifestyle—eating a healthy diet, maintaining a healthy abdominal weight (girth), being physically active for at least thirty minutes
a day, not smoking, and not drinking excessive amounts of alcohol.[30]

- **Predisposition from heredity (genetics).** About one in twenty people
  with colorectal cancer have a well-defined genetic syndrome called
  Lynch Syndrome that is known to predispose individuals with it to
  a type of colorectal cancer called h*ereditary non-polyposis colorectal cancer,* and accounts for 2–4 percent of all diagnosed cases of
  colorectal cancer. It is an autosomal dominant hereditary condition,
  caused by genetic mutations that increase risk for several cancers,
  the highest risk being for colorectal cancer, followed by cancer of
  the endometrium in women. Some estimates place lifetime risk for
  colon cancer among men and women with the Lynch syndrome at
  66 and 43 percent respectively. A diagnosis of colorectal cancer at
  an earlier age (average forty-five years of age) relative to colorectal
  cancer of the non-hereditary type is characteristic of the Lynch
  syndrome. The median age at diagnosis of colon cancer among those
  with the syndrome is reported to be forty-two years for men and
  forty-seven for women.[31] Therefore, a strong family history may
  warrant DNA testing for the gene mutation, and if the results are
  positive, screening by colonoscopy for colorectal cancer beginning
  by age twenty-five or ten years before the age of the youngest
  person in the immediate family was diagnosed with the disease
  is recommended. After the initial colonoscopy, repeating it every

one to two years through age forty, and then annually thereafter is also recommended because once developed, this type of colorectal cancer progresses rapidly.

• **Familial adenomatous polyposis (FAP).** The second most common genetic syndrome is *familial adenomatous polyposis (FAP)*, where one or more family members have been diagnosed with *polyps* (a polyp is a benign tumor with a pedicle, as shown in Figure 6, that sometimes turns into cancer) originating in the glandular tissue. Without detection and removal of the polyps, the lifetime risk of colorectal cancer approaches 100 percent for these individuals.[32]

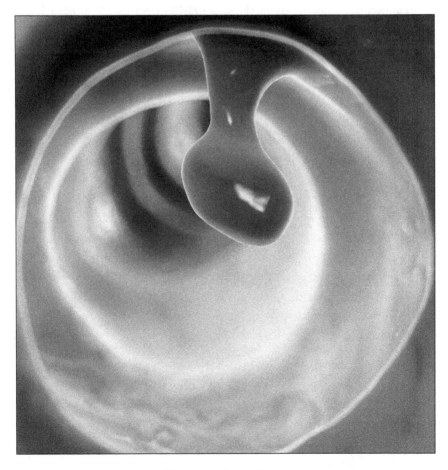

Figure 6. Colon Polyp

- **Family history.** People with a first-degree relative (parent, sibling, or biological child) who has had colorectal cancer have two to three times the risk of developing the disease compared to individuals with no family history. In the U.S., the median age for a diagnosis of colorectal cancer is sixty-eight years in men and seventy-two years in women. If a first-degree relative was diagnosed at a younger age, and if there is more than one affected relative, the risk jumps to three to six times that of the general population.[33] About one in five of those diagnosed with colorectal cancer has a close relative who was also diagnosed with the disease. This underscores the importance of reporting a family history of colorectal cancer to your healthcare provider so it is documented in your medical record, and you can be screened for the disease in a timely manner.

- **Personal medical history.** People who have been diagnosed and treated for colorectal cancer are more likely to develop new cancers in other areas of the colon and rectum, even if the first cancer was completely removed. The risk of a second cancer is known to be greater if the first cancer was diagnosed at age sixty or younger. As well, people who have been diagnosed with one or more adenomatous (benign) polyps have an increased risk of colorectal cancer, especially if the polyps were large or if there was more than one. Individuals, who have a history of chronic inflammatory bowel disease, such as ulcerative colitis or Crohn's disease, where the colon is inflamed, also have an increased risk of developing colorectal cancer, and the risk escalates with the severity and duration of the disease. It is estimated that 18 percent of those with a thirty-year history of ulcerative colitis will likely develop colorectal cancer.[34]

- **Type-2 diabetes.** Multiple studies have reported an association between increased risk for colorectal cancer and type-2 diabetes. The two diseases share some risk factors, physical inactivity and obesity among them, and a positive association between the two diseases persisted in these studies even after accounting for physical activity, body mass index, and waist circumference. One particular study found this association to be stronger in men than in women.[35]

- **Overweight and Obesity.** Both overweight and obesity increase the risk for colorectal cancer and death from it independent of physical activity. And with increasing body mass index (BMI), the association is found to be incremental, indicative of the strength of the association. The link is stronger, and more consistently observed in men than in women. One large cohort study reported the relative risk of death from colorectal cancer among men with a body mass index (BMI) between 35.0 and 39.9 to be 1.8 (risk is 1.8 times that of those with normal weight and average BMI), and 1.4 in women at the corresponding BMI levels. In both men and women, central obesity, reflected by a larger-than-average waist circumference, has been reported to be more of a factor in predicting the risk for colon cancer than overall obesity.[36]

- **Diet.** Differences in colorectal cancer rates across countries and regions, and the changing rates among immigrant populations suggest that diet plays an important role in the risk of developing colorectal cancer, with information on the role of specific dietary elements still being gathered. Several studies, including a large joint study by Harvard University and AARP (American Association of Retired Persons), have found that high consumption of red and/or processed meats increases the risk of both colon and rectal cancer. Evidence from this and other studies also reveals that the risk may be related to cooking meats at high temperatures because a higher risk is observed among those who consume meat cooked at a high temperature for a long period of time. When meat is cooked at high temperatures, chemicals called *heterocyclic* amines, which are known carcinogens, are produced.[37] There is no evidence of any direct association between fat intake and colorectal-cancer risk, but there is evidence that a high-fat diet does increase the risk of developing adenomatous polyps, some of which eventually develop into cancers.[38] Although the evidence is not strong, some studies do suggest that people who eat few fruits and vegetables are also at higher risk for colon cancer.[39] Other studies point to low levels of vitamin D (obtained naturally from sunlight or from nutritional supplements) in blood being associated with an increased risk for colorectal cancer, and the consumption of such calcium-rich foods as milk and other dairy products being associated with a decreased risk.[40]

- Smoking. According to the International Agency for Research on Cancer, there is sufficient empirical evidence that points to a positive association between tobacco smoking and colorectal-cancer risk, with the association being stronger for rectal than colon cancer.[41,42] It is believed that earlier studies may have failed to detect this association because of the long latency period of three to four decades between tobacco exposure and a diagnosis of colorectal cancer.

- Alcohol consumption. The risk for colorectal cancer has been associated with even moderate alcohol use. On average, individuals who have two to four alcoholic drinks per day were found to have a 23-percent higher risk of colorectal cancer than those who consume less than one drink per day on average.[43]

- Medications. There is sufficient evidence suggesting that long-term, regular use of aspirin and other non-steroidal anti-inflammatory drugs (NSAIDS) is associated with a lower risk of colorectal cancer.[44] However, the potential side effects of gastrointestinal bleeding from aspirin and similar drugs do not warrant their use for cancer prevention. Those who are already taking these for chronic arthritis, or low-dose aspirin for heart-disease prevention, may experience a lower risk of colorectal cancer as an additional benefit.

- Hormone therapy. Many studies have found that women who use postmenopausal hormone therapy have lower rates of colorectal cancer than those who do not.[45] A decreased risk is especially evident in women with long-term hormone use, and they are shown to return to pre-hormone-therapy risk levels within three years of discontinuing the therapy. However, prominent studies, such as the Women's Health Initiative Study, also found that the use of postmenopausal hormone therapy, especially the combination hormone therapy, increases the risk for breast and other cancers, as well as cardiovascular disease. Therefore, hormone therapy is not specifically recommended for the prevention of colorectal cancer. In general, given the uncertainties about their effectiveness, appropriate dose, and potential toxicity, the American Cancer Society does not recommend any medications to prevent colorectal cancer.

THE NATURAL HISTORY OF COLORECTAL CANCER

While all cancers have a long latency period between risk exposure and development of the disease, a particularly long latency period of three to four decades seems to be characteristic of colorectal cancer. The unusually long latency period explains, at least in part, the higher median age (sixty-eight years in men and seventy-two years in women) for a diagnosis of colorectal cancers in the U.S. The susceptibility to colorectal cancer begins with exposure to one or more of the risk factors described above. The earliest detectable indicator of a possible impending cancer of the colon or rectum is the presence of one or more polyps, which, if left to remain, may turn cancerous. The polyps are detected by the available screening tests, such as flexible sigmoidoscopy

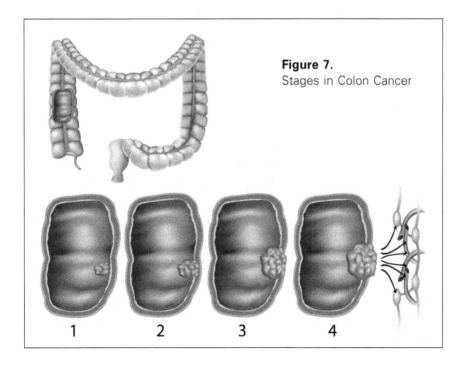

Figure 7.
Stages in Colon Cancer

1   2   3   4

and colonoscopy. These tests are recommended starting at age fifty, and repeating at intervals dictated by the initial test results and the individual risk level, ranging between three to ten years on average. Cancerous tumors and some large polyps bleed intermittently into the intestine, with the blood finding its way into the stool. However, since the small amount of blood is undetectable to the naked eye, it is referred to as occult blood. A test called fecal occult blood test (FOBT) can detect very small quantities of blood in the stool, and an FOBT kit for use at home can be obtained from a healthcare provider or the lab.

Colorectal tumors and large polyps also shed cells into the large bowel that contain altered DNA (gene mutations). These abnormal cellular changes are detectable with the use of a DNA stool test, such as the sDNA test that detects gene mutations in stool samples. As with FOBT, a test kit can be obtained from a healthcare provider or the lab for specimen collection at home. Studies have shown that the regular use of these simple, easy-to-do screening methods reduces the risk of death from colorectal cancer by 15–33 percent.[46]

PREVENTION OF COLORECTAL CANCER

The primary prevention of colorectal cancer is targeted at avoiding or minimizing exposure to modifiable risk factors—overweight and obesity, red-meat consumption (especially cooked at high temperatures), smoking, and alcohol consumption. Early detection and surgical removal of polyps is also an important step in preventing colorectal cancer and averting the transition from polyp to cancer. Getting screened at the recommended age and correct intervals goes a long way in detecting pre-cancerous polyps and also capturing probable cases of cancer early, before it has a chance to spread to other parts of the body, is easier to treat, and adds a significantly better prognosis for cure and survival. There are currently a number of screening tests that can be used as preliminary tools prior to the use of more definitive diagnostic methods like a biopsy to confirm cancer. Currently, twenty-six states and the District of Columbia have enacted laws requiring private insurers to cover the full range of colorectal-cancer screening tests for all individuals at the appropriate age and intervals.

THE STORY OF JOE, THE OPTIMIST

Joe, a fifty-seven-year-old man, first came to see me with the complaints of generalized abdominal symptoms—bloating, cramps, mild diarrhea, and heartburn. He had recently returned from visiting his extended family in Central America, and said he might have eaten something there that made him sick. He denied having fever, chills, night sweats, headache, vomiting, or loosing weight. Joe did not appear ill, and all his vital signs were normal. However, he did seem anxious, and when asked, said his mother was dying from colon cancer. His exam, including his abdomen, did not reveal anything out of the ordinary. His abdomen was not distended, was not tender to touch, and he had normal bowel sounds. He had no enlargement of any internal organs, and no palpable mass. I asked Joe to submit a sample of his stool to the laboratory to check for any infection; the results came back negative, and after a few days his symptoms improved.

Three weeks later, Joe returned to my office with an exacerbation of the same abdominal symptoms he had experienced earlier. Again, he did not report having any other symptoms, such as fever, chills, night sweats, headaches, vomiting, or weight loss, suggestive of something serious or systemic. His physical examination also turned out normal, but this time I performed a digital rectal exam and tested a small sample of his stool under the microscope. The result was positive for blood in the stool. There were several plausible explanations for the blood in Joe's stool, such as an irritated bowel from his recent diarrhea, irritated internal hemorrhoids, or because he was still experiencing stress over his mother's illness and had developed a silent peptic ulcer. I sent Joe to the lab for blood tests. The results showed that he had mild anemia with hemoglobin of 11.5 g/dL (normal range; 13.5–18 g/dL) and his ESR (erythrocyte sedimentation rate) was slightly elevated, which is a sign of inflammation in the body. This meant that Joe had probably been gradually losing blood through his gastrointestinal tract for some time, or he might have developed inflammatory bowel disease. He was referred to a gastroenterologist for further evaluation.

The gastroenterologist evaluated Joe, had additional blood and stool tests done, and scheduled him for an upper endoscopy and colonoscopy.

The blood and stool tests came up negative, but his endoscopy revealed a small area of gastric erosion with moderate inflammation of his duodenum (the beginning of the small intestine). The colonoscopy showed a large non-obstructing mass in his ascending (right) colon, and a 15mm polyp in his sigmoid (left) colon, both of which were more ominous (possible cancer) than the gastric erosion. The sigmoid polyp was snared and removed entirely and the large mass was biopsied and tattooed (marked) for identification during possible surgery later. The pathology results suggested that the mass in his colon could be adenocarcinoma (cancer), and the polyp could be a benign (non-cancerous) tubular adenoma. A CT scan was then ordered of his chest, abdomen, and pelvis. The scan showed a 6-centimeter mass in the mid ascending colon, highly suggestive of cancer and a possible local metastasis (spread) to adjacent lymph nodes. There was no evidence of spread of cancer to his lungs, liver, or pelvic organs. Joe was operated on a few days later, and underwent a laparoscopic-assisted right colectomy. Forty-three regional lymph nodes were removed along with the cancer mass and were tested for the presence of cancer, but none showed any cancer spread. Following surgery, a medical-oncology consultation was obtained. Based on the facts that Joe was fifty-seven-years-old at the time of his diagnosis and the just-removed cancerous mass was significantly large, the medical oncologist determined that he was a candidate for chemotherapy. Joe completed twelve cycles of chemotherapy and tolerated it reasonably well. Further tests showed no evidence of any cancer spread and no new tumor growth.

Since Joe's mother had also been diagnosed with colon cancer when she turned eighty, additional tests were performed to determine if Joe's cancer was consistent with Lynch syndrome, an inherited colon-cancer syndrome, but there was no strong evidence of this in the tests, which meant Joe's estimated risk of recurring cancer is no higher than 13 to 15 percent. It's been four years since he was first diagnosed with colon cancer, and to date Joe's colonoscopies have been negative for additional polyps or cancer. Joe remains optimistic, and says he takes one day at a time and tries to make the best of each day. His positive outlook and his supportive family seem to be his best assets in the battle with cancer.

SAM'S FIFTIETH BIRTHDAY PRESENT TO HIMSELF

Sam is a fifty-two-year-old man who has been a patient of mine for some years. Just after turning fifty, he came in for a physical examination. Sam was already being treated for hypertension, mixed dyslipidemia, and obstructive sleep apnea, for which he had undergone oral surgery several years before. He is 6' tall and weighed 208 pounds, with a BMI of 28 (a BMI between 25 and 29 is considered overweight). Sam's health history revealed that he had chewed tobacco for thirty years. On the day of his visit, his blood pressure was 128/88 mmHg, an indication that his BP was being reasonably controlled with treatment.

Sam had some blood tests, and was given a kit for stool test (FIT) to detect any occult (hidden) blood in the stool in an amount that is not detectable by the naked eye. He was referred for a screening colonoscopy as he just had his fiftieth birthday. When his test results came back, I went over the results with Sam and explained what each of them meant. His cholesterol levels were slightly higher than the desired levels, but more importantly his stool test was positive for blood. This meant that somewhere in his gastrointestinal tract, Sam was bleeding, but in such a small amount that it is not seen by the naked eye, but detectable by the stool test. Since Sam had not yet scheduled an appointment for a colonoscopy, I reiterated the importance of doing so as soon as possible, especially in light of his positive stool test. I gave him a copy of his stool test results indicating the presence of occult blood, and told him I would also be sending the results to the gastroenterologist I referred him to.

About two months later, Sam had his colonoscopy, which revealed a 3–4 cm mass attached to the wall of his cecum (the beginning of his right colon). He also had a 1 cm polyp further down his colon on the left side. The polyp was removed in its entirety, and during the procedure several tissue samples were taken from the mass in his cecum. Pathology results of these biopsies showed a high-grade dysplasia (abnormal cells) in both tumors. A CT scan of his abdomen and pelvis, were done to rule out metastatic disease, but showed no evidence of any spread. Shortly thereafter, Sam underwent a laparoscopic (reaching into the abdomen through small incisions) right colectomy that removed the tumor, and adjacent lymph nodes. The pathology test of the tumor revealed a well-differentiated adenocarcinoma (malignant tumor) of the cecum, but there was no evidence of any spread to the adjacent lymph nodes or vasculature—the lymph nodes that were removed along with the malignant tumor were all negative for evidence of cancer spread. Because the cancer was found early, the medical oncologist determined that Sam did not require chemotherapy post surgery.

A follow-up colonoscopy one year later revealed a small 3mm polyp in Sam's sigmoid colon that was removed during the procedure. Biopsy results affirmed that the polyp was a benign (non-cancerous) tubular adenoma. Because Sam was fifty years of age when he developed colon cancer, he received genetic counseling for a possible hereditary cancer syndrome—the Lynch syndrome (an autosomal dominant predisposition to colon cancer). The geneticist determined that Sam's particular cancer was a sporadic event, not an inherited mutation associated with Lynch syndrome.

Sam continues to be monitored closely for any changes in his status. His case underscores the importance of doing both the stool test for occult blood when advised, and the screening colonoscopy at age fifty or earlier if there is a family history of colon cancer. In his case, the early detection of his colon cancer and the prompt surgical treatment helped save his life, by stopping the further progression and spread of his cancer. So Sam gave himself the best birthday present of all by having the colposcopy when advised. His use of smokeless tobacco, however, is a lifestyle choice he would have been better off without because tobacco use, even the smokeless kind, is associated with an increased risk for certain types of cancers.

7

Obesity

In recent years, obesity has been classified as a chronic disease. The World Health organization (WHO) defines obesity as body mass index (BMI) of 30 or more and a condition of excess body fat to the extent that health is impaired.[1] Obesity, like other chronic diseases described earlier, is a progressive disease, often developed over many years. And, like other chronic health conditions, it too has a long latency period—many of those diagnosed with obesity are young adults (mid-thirties) and most of the associated long-term harmful health consequences do not surface until sometime, often years, later. This long latency has the effect of lulling people with the disease into believing they are healthy now and will continue to be so in the future. Numerous studies have shown, however, that obesity increases the risk of developing other chronic diseases, such as type-2 diabetes, heart disease, and certain cancers.[2] Following tobacco use, obesity has become the second leading preventable cause of disease and death in the United States.[3]

The prevalence of overweight and obesity is increasing globally. According to the National Center for Health Statistics (NCHS), the most recent national data on obesity among U.S. adults, adolescents, and children show that more than one-third of adults (36 percent) and just over 18 percent of children and adolescents between the ages of six and nineteen years were obese in 2011–2012.[4] The rate of obesity was higher among boys than girls (18.6 vs.15.0 percent). Even very young children between the ages of two and five years are not escaping obesity, as 12 percent of them are also obese. These numbers reflect an increase of more than 25 percent in obesity over the past three decades. Obesity is defined in terms of body mass index (BMI), which is calculated by dividing weight in kilograms by height in meters squared, rounded to one decimal place (if using the non-metric system, divide the weight in pounds by height in inches squared and multiply by a conversion factor of 703). Normal weight is regarded as being between BMI 18.5 and 24.9, and is the same for men and women. Those with BMI between 25 and 29.9 are considered overweight, and those with BMI 30 or greater are labeled obese. For diagnostic purposes, obesity is further divided into different grades as follows:

- Grade I (BMI 30-34.9);

- Grade II (BMI 35-39.9);

- Grade III (BMI 40 and greater). This category of obesity is sometimes referred to as morbid, or severe, obesity.

Obesity is a risk factor for many chronic conditions, including type-2 diabetes, hypertension, high cholesterol, stroke, heart disease, some cancers, osteoarthritis, sleep apnea, and depression. The health risks associated with severe form of obesity (BMI of 40 or greater) are greater because the individuals in this category are more likely to develop multiple disease conditions, known in medical terminology as *co-morbidities.* Although trends in health outcomes in obesity-related conditions do not always parallel trends in obesity rates, in part due to improvements in diagnosis and treatment, many deaths from cardiovascular disease, diabetes, and certain cancers are associated with the condition.

In recent years, some have challenged the assumption that obesity is universally associated with higher death rates.Some studies have even reported an inverse relationship between obesity and mortality (the death rate) in selected other diseases, including heart failure, coronary artery disease, and kidney failure.[5] This seemingly paradoxical and controversial finding has garnered much publicity and generated an interest in further exploration of the association. Ensuing research yielded inconsistent results that neither validated the challenge, nor refuted it altogether. Two large studies, one from each camp, are noteworthy. In one large pooled analysis of prospective studies comprising 1.4 million white adult participants, both overweight and obesity were found to be associated with increased all-cause mortality. The lowest all-cause mortality in this study was generally observed in the BMI range of 20.0 to 24.9.[6] A second study examined the association between BMI and mortality in 2.9 million people, among whom there were 270,000 deaths during the study period. They found that while the more severe forms of obesity (grades II and III) were associated with significantly higher all-cause mortality, grade I obesity (BMI 30 to 34.9) was not, and overweight (BMI 25 to 29.9) was, in-fact, associated with *reduced* mortality. This led them to conclude that overweight, and mild obesity may have a protective effect that extends the lifespan. Rather than put the controversy to rest, this and similar claims gave rise to skepticism and led to speculation within the scientific community about possible alternate explanations for the findings. One plausible alternative offered for the inverse relationship of even mild obesity to mortality is that the healthcare providers may be targeting obese individuals for more aggressive diagnostic and treatment strategies than normal weight individuals, leading to better health outcomes and lower mortality among them. Another, rival hypothesis for the finding led to questioning the use of BMI to define obesity, which many agree does not precisely measure body-fat content or reflect the proportion of muscle to fat. One other criticism of BMI as a measure of body mass is that it does not account for gender and racial differences in fat content or for the distribution of visceral (abdominal) and subcutaneous fat. These criticisms have led some to propose the body-shape index (ABSI), which measures abdominal fat as a better predictor of mortality than BMI, as excessive visceral fat, is associated with the previously described metabolic syndrome. The BMI, however, remains the most practical and widely used measure to evaluate the degree of overweight as it correlates well with body fat and provides a standardized definition of obesity for the purposes of national and international comparisons. The National Institutes of Health in the U.S. and the World Health Organization (WHO) have both endorsed the use of BMI for uniform definitions of overweight and obesity. The fact that obesity is associated with several chronic diseases that are responsible for a majority of deaths in the U.S. remains undisputed.

The trends and patterns of the increasing prevalence of overweight and obesity across the age, gender, racial, and ethnic groups, and the associated negative impact on public health warrant an urgent and multi-pronged approach to preventing or reducing their occurrence. In January 2013, The American Medical Association (AMA) officially recognized obesity as a chronic disease—the World Health Organization had done so much earlier. Being formally defined as a disease, obesity should spur healthcare providers, patients, and health insurers alike to regard it as a serious medical condition that requires intervention. Many in the healthcare field agree that due to its negative impact on public health, obesity is one of the greatest threats to health in the current era.[7] Obesity also adds substantially to the already skyrocketing healthcare costs, a fact that prompted a sitting U.S. President to raise concern over it in his State of the Union address to the joint congress on January 28, 2014.

RISK FACTORS FOR OBESITY

The unprecedented rise in the prevalence of obesity in recent decades involves a complex interaction among genetic, socioeconomic, demographic, environmental, and lifestyle factors. As mentioned, obesity is a progressive disease, often spanning many years and stages from normal weight, to overweight, to obese states, and several gradations within those stages. Although its causes are complex, the overarching, underlying, direct cause of obesity is a greater consumption of energy than is used by the body. Many agree that a host of social and environmental factors might have a profound effect on influencing lifestyles that enable the high consumption and low expenditure of energy patterns, and are fueling the obesity epidemic in the United States and worldwide. A new term, *obesogenic*, has even been coined to describe the prevailing societal environment in the United States that can be characterized by its promotion of a high-energy intake and a low-energy expenditure. Americans have access to an abundance of low-cost (not necessarily healthy) food, and there are plenty of energy-saving opportunities at work and home that facilitate sedentary behaviors throughout the day. Within this environment, however, there are many factors affecting the energy intake and expenditure phenomenon that promote obesity, the most influential being age, sex, race or ethnicity, and socioeconomic status (SES). Obesity's associations with these factors are dynamic and complex, and an understanding of the dynamics involved not only helps healthcare providers identify those at risk for obesity and target them for early intervention, but also helps those in the *at-risk* groups, as well as their loved ones, to be aware of the undesirable influences around them and guard against them.

The Age Factor

The influence of age in developing obesity is gathered from studying population trends over time and capturing the age range when obesity becomes prevalent. From these studies, it is apparent that, throughout early adulthood, the average body mass index (BMI) increases with age. The data from these studies reveal that, while obesity rates doubled for adults in the past three decades, the rates for adolescents tripled during the same period. It is also evident from these data that, during their lifetime, younger individuals are experiencing a longer (cumulative) exposure to obesity and the associated risks from it.[8] Analyses of obesity trends in the U.S. also show a second weight trend, reflecting a tendency among those born in the later calendar years to have larger age-specific BMI values. The findings point to a two-year increment in the birth year being linked with a more rapid onset of obesity, reflecting a progressively earlier onset of obesity. It is also evident from the data analysis that fewer than 15 percent of those who were mildly or moderately obese at age twenty to twenty-two years were free from obesity at age thirty-five to thirty-seven years, suggesting that although obesity can be reversed, it is uncommon. This was found to be true in all racial and ethnic groups, and warrants targeting obesity-prevention efforts at those just transitioning into adulthood who exhibit any level of overweight.

Race, Ethnicity, and Gender Differences

The influence of race and gender on obesity seems to be more complex than the age factor. Race and gender, alone and in combination, appear to exert different influences on obesity, and these are revealed in a comprehensive review of obesity trends, based on nationally representative data obtained from studies published between 1990 and 2006. In both genders, non-Hispanic blacks and Hispanic adults are reported to have the highest rate of obesity. Black women had the highest average BMI values, and white women had the lowest. The prevalence of extreme obesity (BMI 40 or greater) is also reported to be higher among black women relative to other groups. Both black and Hispanic women tend to reach obesity at a younger age than white women. The average BMI reached overweight status in black women by age twenty-six, in Hispanic women by age twenty-eight, and in white women by age thirty-five.[9]

Men also showed race-based differences in average BMIs. Both black and white men show similar rates of obesity onset at the transition into adulthood, but obesity develops more rapidly in black men after twenty-eight years of age. Hispanic men, however, consistently had the highest mean age-specific BMI values. The average BMI reached overweight status by age twenty-five in Hispanic men and by age twenty-seven in all other men. Hispanic ethnicity appears associated with the most rapid onset of obesity at all ages. The other racial groups with high rates of obesity include Native Americans and Pacific Islanders. The prevalence of obesity is significantly lower among Asian Americans than among other racial/ethnic groups, 5 percent versus 30 percent. Adjusted for race or ethnicity, childhood weight development, and birth year, women overall are twice as likely as men to become obese by ages thirty-five to thirty-seven. This underscores the importance of targeting women for obesity prevention before they reach the age of thirty-five. It has been suggested that race, ethnicity, and gender are likely surrogates for such other factors as dietary and exercise standards, income, and education.

Socioeconomic Status (SES)

At all ages, minority and low socioeconomic status (SES) groups are disproportionately affected by obesity. In the U.S. the patterns of obesity in children, adolescents, and adults have some similarities among them, but some features are unique to a specific age group. Socioeconomic status is inversely related to the rate of obesity among whites, but not to the same extent among African-Americans or Hispanics. Studies based on data gathered in the National Health and Nutrition Examination Surveys (NHANES) of a nationally representative sample of Americans have shown that young boys from higher SES families had the lowest levels of obesity compared with their counterparts from lower SES families, but such a disparity was small among young girls.[10] Among adolescent boys, there was no consistent association found between SES and overweight, but adolescent girls from lower SES backgrounds had a much higher rate of overweight than their middle- and high-SES counterparts (20.0 vs. 14.2 and 12 percent, respectively). This pattern appears especially true among white adolescent girls, whereas black adolescent girls from higher SES families were at an increased risk for obesity compared to their lower-SES counterparts (38.0 vs. 18.7 and 24.5 percent respectively). The NHANES data show that, with the exception of black women, those with less than a high school education in the United States have an overall higher obesity rate than their counterparts with a high school or higher education. Black women with less than a high school education had the lowest rate compared to those who had higher educational levels, so there do not appear to be any consistent patterns for an SES difference in the rising rates of obesity.

A growing number of studies have revealed the complexity of the relationship between gender, ethnicity, socioeconomic status (SES), and obesity among U.S. adults since the late 1980s. Researchers have noted that the association between SES and obesity varies by ethnicity, and that racial differences in BMI are not fully explained by SES alone. They point out that ethnic/racial differentials in BMI may, instead, be explained by contributing factors, such as body image, lifestyle, and social and physical environments that are conceptually distinct from

SES. Neither education nor income, two commonly used components of SES, equally reflect the association with obesity across ethnic groups. They also suggest there may be a two-way causal relation between SES and obesity, because obesity may adversely affect opportunities for education, occupation, and marriage.

Time and Geographic Trends

Based on the available national data, the Centers for Disease Control and Prevention reported that 35 percent of U.S. adults were obese (BMI of 30 or greater) in 2010. The obesity rate in the United States increased steadily, but at a slower pace between 1960 and 1980, but after 1980, it increased dramatically, doubling between 1976 and 2000 from 15.1 to 30.9 percent. The annual rate of increase was similar for men and women during this period. There does not appear to be any slowing or even a leveling off in the rate of increase of obesity in recent years.[10,11]

The regional differences in the rates of overweight and obesity became apparent over time, especially between 1990 and 2005. In 1990, none of the fifty states in the U.S. had obesity rates at or above 20 percent, and only five had a rate between 15 and 19 percent. In 1995, the Western and Northeastern states were registering a lower prevalence (10–14 percent) than states in other regions (15–19 percent). By the year 2000, thirty-two of the fifty states had obesity rates of 20 percent or higher, and the burden of obesity started shifting toward Southern and Eastern states. In 2005, only four states had obesity rates of 20 percent or lower, while twenty-six states ranged between a rate of 20 and 25, seventeen states reported a rate of 25 percent or more, and three states had a rate of 30 percent or more. The regional variation in the rate of childhood obesity is substantial with the South-Central region registering the highest (18 percent), and the Mountain Region the lowest (11.4 percent). A national survey of children found that children in West Virginia, Kentucky, Texas, Tennessee, and North Carolina were twice as likely to be obese as children of the same age and gender in Utah.[11] The survey revealed that individual characteristics, such as race, ethnicity, socioeconomic status of the household, television viewing, recreational computer use, and physical activity, accounted for a substantial portion of the variation in childhood obesity (55 percent variation between states; 25 percent between regions). This points to the fact that social and environmental factors are intertwined with geographic location, and play an important role in causing childhood obesity, and thus should be taken into account when targeting prevention efforts.

Genetics

Since the recent unprecedented rise in overweight and obesity cannot be explained by changes in the human gene pool, the scientific community has come to accept the fact that environmental factors play the most important role in the development of overweight and obesity. Even so, there do seem to be lingering questions about the role of genetics in the cause of obesity, and in recent years there has been a significant amount of research and a growing body of knowledge about the genetics behind obesity. The genes responsible for obesity in mice have been identified, and the mechanisms behind the control of body-fat accumulation have been recognized, at least in part. It has been hypothesized by genetics researchers that obesity genes may be involved in the regulation of human adipose-tissue function, and might cause excess body fat by a direct interaction with the adipose (fat) cell.[12] Results from genomic scans suggest that major obesity genes are located on chromosomes 2, 10, 11, and 20, and researchers have suggested that these chromosomes contain one or several genes that may play a role in the control of body weight. The strength of the association with obesity for each individual gene is relatively weak; some are believed to be important for obesity only among women. Genetic factors are believed to be responsible for fat distribution in the body, and since fat is distributed differently in men and women, it is suggested that men and women may have different obesity genes.

There has long been a search for a genetic cause of rare forms of obesity. Using recent developments in DNA technology, families with a juvenile onset of extreme obesity have been screened for mutations in the genes that have been found to cause obesity in mice, but to date the results have come up negative in humans. The mechanisms responsible for excess fat accumulation in rare forms of human obesity are not yet known. Researchers also acknowledge that the genetics involved in common forms of human obesity are not yet well understood. An emerging science, *molecular pathological epidemiology*, has been successful in its approach to the study of cancers, and offers future promise for investigating subtypes of obesity that might reveal more about the precise role of genetics in obesity. In the meantime it might not be in the interest of those affected by obesity to believe that genetics may be responsible for their excess weight gain as it may keep them from even trying to reverse their disease. After all, in the vast majority of cases, it is the energy imbalance (taking in more and expending less) and not genetics that is responsible for excess weight gain.

Hormones

One of the many functions of hormones in the body is to regulate metabolism, including fat metabolism. Insulin, a hormone typically associated with diabetes, is believed to play a key role in the development of obesity. Insulin is important in both *lipogenesis* (fat formation), and inhibition of *lipolysis* (decomposition of fat). Destruction of the pancreatic (beta) cells in experimental animals has shown to slow or arrest the development of obesity. A lack of sufficient insulin production, as seen in type-1 diabetes, is associated with normal body weight, whereas overweight is often, if not always, associated with type-2 diabetes, when the body's cells can't use insulin effectively or the pancreas can't make enough insulin to keep up with an increasing demand. Thyroid hormones influence your heart rate, basal metabolic rate, body weight, and various aspects of fat, carbohydrate, protein, and mineral metabolism. The thyroid hormone is also regarded as an important determinant of overall energy expenditure and the regulation of body temperature through thermogenesis (heat generation). Abnormally low or high thyroid hormones are associated with weight gain or loss respectively. Both are easily treatable conditions and do not account for any significant weight gain or loss beyond transitory periods. Although increased thyroid levels can reduce fat and thus improve cholesterol levels, harmful effects on the heart, muscle, and bone counterbalance these positive effects. For this reason, the use of thyroid hormones for cholesterol-lowering and weight loss purposes is not recommended.[13]

Both male (androgens) and female (estrogens) hormones are involved in fat distribution and obesity. And after puberty, the production of testosterone in men is associated with a reduction in the percentage of body fat that makes it possible to achieve the six-pack abdomen so sought after by young men. After reaching puberty, the increase in estrogen is involved in producing the female shaped body that reflects fat distribution differently from that of their male counterparts. When ovaries are surgically removed in animals, obesity frequently develops, and can be reversed by giving injections of estrogen. Many of the cancers associated with obesity—cancer of the breast, prostate, endometrium, colon, and gallbladder—are known to have a hormonal basis. In overweight postmenopausal women, an increase in the production of estrogenic compounds has been linked to the amount of fat in the body. While this may provide an important source of estrogen for the postmenopausal woman, it may also increase their risk for developing endometrial and breast cancer.[14] Experimental mice lacking *gastrin* (a hormone secreted by the mucosal lining of the stomach) become obese and exhibit an increased risk of developing colon cancer, a deadly disease in humans if not detected and treated in its early stage.

Environmental Factors

Evidence to date points to the fact that the current obesity epidemic is largely caused by an environment that promotes excessive food intake, but does not encourage or necessitate physical activity to expend it, leading to an energy imbalance. A wide range of factors—increasing urbanization, economic growth, increasing availability of calorie-dense sweeteners and other processed convenience foods, an increase in the frequency of eating out, and innovations in technology—all working in concert have contributed to a rising incidence of overweight and obesity in many Western countries, but in the U.S. the same is occurring in a precipitous and pronounced way. Some scientists theorize that during famines and other periods of diminished food supply, human physiological mechanisms have evolved to protect against severe weight loss, but comparable physiological mechanisms have not evolved to defend against body weight gain when food is abundant.[15] Behaviors that protect against obesity include control of portion sizes, consumption of a diet low in fat and energy density, and regular physical activity, but in the current environment, there are many challenges to adopting and maintaining these behaviors.

Beginning in the last decades of the twentieth century and continuing into the twenty-first, major shifts in dietary patterns, characterized by a high intake of saturated fats, sugar, refined foods, and low fiber, coupled with lower levels of physical activity patterns, seemed to parallel a rise in prevalence of overweight and obesity in the U.S. Several trends and patterns in energy consumption, such as an increased consumption of total energy—soft drinks, calorie-dense snack foods, more frequent eating at fast-food and other restaurants—and not eating adequate amounts of recommended vegetables and fruits seemed to have placed people in the United States at a greatly increased risk for obesity. Plus, over the past three decades, the increased size of portions served is also likely an important contributor to the overconsumption of food, and many say this has fueled the growing obesity epidemic in the U.S.[16]

Of particular concern are those foods that have a too-high energy density. Studies have found that large portions of the energy-dense foods lead to excess energy intake, and contribute to obesity. This observation has been supported by data collected in many settings, and across many population groups. Trends in food-portion sizes show that they began to grow in the 1970s, rose sharply in the 1980s, and are continuing to parallel increased body weights. In recent decades, the supersizing of portions served in restaurants, the fast food kind in particular, with only a minimal additional cost, is also likely an important contributor to the overconsumption of food, and many say this has fueled the growing obesity epidemic in the U.S.[16] The increase in both portion size and the frequency of eating away from home have paralleled the rising rates of obesity in the U.S. Portion sizes for foods and beverages are also associated with childhood obesity. Among U.S. children ages two to eighteen years, some alarming trends in food-portion sizes and the association with total meal sizes were shown in four nationally representative surveys of food intake between 1977–1978 and 2003–2006. One trend points to an increase in energy derived from selected key foods—soft/fruit drinks, salty snacks, desserts, French fries, burgers, pizzas, Mexican fast foods, and hot dogs—totaling a quarter of the total energy consumed.[17]

The increased consumption of caloric sweeteners is one of the dietary changes worldwide, and it is reflected by a small but consistent increase in energy intake between 1962 and 2000. In the U.S., caloric sweeteners represented a 22-percent increase in the proportion of energy supplied by sweeteners during this period. The largest portion (80 percent) of this increase comes from sugared beverages, while the remaining percentage is contributed by restaurant and fast food sources. It has been reported that the consumption of one particular caloric sweetener, high-fructose corn syrup (HFCS), has increased more than 1000 percent in the U.S. between 1970 and 1990, and has mirrored the steady rise in overweight and obesity.[18] High-fructose corn syrup now represents over 40 percent of the caloric sweeteners added to foods and beverages, and is currently the primary caloric sweetener in soft drinks in the United States. A conservative estimate shows that Americans two years of age and over consume a daily average of 132 kilocalories from HFCS, and the top 20 percent of those who consume caloric sweeteners take in 316 calories a day from HFCS. The digestion, absorption, and metabolism of fructose differ from those of glucose. The metabolism of fructose results in *lipogenesis* (fat production) in the liver, and, unlike glucose, fructose does not stimulate insulin secretion or enhance *leptin* production (both help regulate food intake and body weight), thus contributing to increased energy intake and weight gain.

Snacking between meals has also been associated with an excess of energy intake and obesity. An increase in eating energy-dense salty snacks and energy beverages, both in amount and frequency, has been reported in all adults from 1977–1978 to 2003–2006. In both men and women, energy intake has been found to increase with snacking frequency irrespective of physical activity, and is noted to be markedly higher in obese individuals. The middle-age group (forty to fifty-nine years) accounted for the highest number of snacks per day in 2003–2006, but those older than sixty experienced the highest increase in the number of snacks per day throughout the 1977–2006 time period. The largest increase in the kilocalories consumed per snacking event between 1977–1978 and 2003–2006 was noted, however, in the younger age group (nineteen to thirty-nine years). Researchers have noted not only major increases in snacking, but also changes in the food sources for snacks over the past decades, with a reported major shift toward an increased intake of salty snacks, chips, and nuts, along with smaller shifts toward reduced amounts of desserts, dairy products, and fruit. The total contribution of calories from snacks to overall calories consumed increased to nearly one quarter between 2003 and 2006. This pattern of snacking among adults has led researchers to conclude that increased snacking may be associated with a greater risk of energy imbalance, and the consequent rise in overweight and obesity.[19]

Physical Inactivity

Incontrovertible evidence links obesity to multiple health problems, including the risk for cardiovascular disease, type-2 diabetes, certain cancers, and all-cause mortality. A rise in the prevalence of obesity appears to be paralleled by decreases in physical activity worldwide, and is consistently found in studies done in the U.S. In observational studies, both overweight and obesity are correlated with physical activity and cardiorespiratory fitness, and data from controlled clinical trials have shown that increases in physical activity result in weight loss and changes in body composition and fat distribution. In one particular study, researchers sought to answer the question of the relationship between physical activity and obesity, fitness, and health.[20] They observed that physical inactivity has a consistent relationship to health outcomes, as does obesity, and that both obesity and inactivity have similar patterns of association with clinical risk indicators, such as blood pressure, fasting plasma glucose, and inflammatory markers. Furthermore, they noted that the association between physical activity and health outcomes is direct and incremental. The researchers also pointed out that the association is biologically plausible, supporting the hypothesis that more physical activity results in better health. Based on their observations, they concluded that declines in average daily energy expenditure are likely an underlying cause of the obesity epidemic in the U.S., allowing the inference that some, perhaps much, of the overweight and obesity seen in the U.S. population is caused by a sedentary, physically inactive lifestyle.

The fact that the amount of physical activity, at least in part, is associated with the physical environment surrounding a person's place of residence is often mentioned in the context of environmental influences on health. A large study done in and around Atlanta, Georgia, to evaluate the relationship between the environment around people's place of residence, the self-reported travel patterns (walking and time spent in a car), and obesity revealed some interesting findings.[21] Measures of the mix of land use, residential density, and street connectivity were recorded within a 1-kilometer network distance of each participant's place of residence. To minimize bias, objective measures of BMI, minutes spent in a car, kilometers walked, age, income, educational attainment, and gender were also obtained from the participants. The land-use mix showed the strongest association with obesity (BMI of 30 or higher), with each quartile increase being associated with a 12.2-percent reduction in obesity, regardless of the gender or ethnicity of the participants. Each additional hour spent in a car per day was associated with a 6-percent increase in the likelihood of obesity. Conversely, each additional kilometer walked per day was associated with a 4.8 percent reduction in the likelihood of obesity. Based on the evidence, the researchers concluded that relationships among the environment and travel patterns are important predictors of obesity across gender and ethnicity. The implication here is to develop strategies to increase land-use mix (increase walking distance, reduce driving distance) to help prevent obesity and reduce the obesity rates.

In the U.K., some interesting accounts of occupation-related activity and chronic disease have come from studies done with London transit workers, postal service employees, and civil servants. One of the earliest such studies found that bus conductors on London's double-decker omnibuses were at lower risk for coronary heart disease than the bus drivers. Even when the conductors did develop the disease, it was less severe, and they were more likely to survive a heart attack than the drivers. The researchers attributed the differential to the conductors constantly being on their feet, moving about, and going up and down the stairs of the double-decker buses. Another eight-year study of British civil servants also reported a two-fold difference in mortality rates of those who reported some kind of vigorous exercise (death rate was 4.2 per 1000) and those who did not report any vigorous exercise (8.4 per 1000). The difference persisted even when factors of age, smoking, and obesity were taken into account. These studies illustrate the fact that physical activity of either high intensity (vigorous exercise) or low-to-moderate intensity (walking and stair climbing) has health benefits.[22]

Research strongly suggests that exercise is a critical component of any program for weight control and health improvement, with even modest levels of physical activity proving sufficient to achieve the weight and health benefits of exercise. For some, the health improvement attained from increased physical activity may be independent of weight loss. In studies, active, fit individuals are consistently shown to have lower rates of morbidity and mortality than sedentary and physically unfit individuals. So, it can be inferred that the higher levels of physical activity or cardiorespiratory fitness do reduce the risk of morbidity and mortality in overweight or obese individuals who are active and fit. They have been shown to have morbidity and mortality rates that are at least as low, and in many instances much lower than normal-weight individuals who are sedentary. These individuals who are active and fit are less likely to develop obesity-related chronic diseases and die from them than those of normal weight individuals who lead sedentary lives. As predictors of disease and death, inactivity and low cardiorespiratory fitness appear to be as important as overweight or obesity.

THE NATURAL HISTORY OF THE DISEASE OF OBESITY

Susceptibility to Obesity

Although the susceptibility to obesity spans age, sex, race, ethnicity, and socioeconomic groups, its age of onset and rate of progression do differ among certain groups. Like other chronic diseases, obesity is also a progressive disease, with incremental gains in body weight. Similar to other chronic diseases, the causes of obesity are complex and encompass a wide range of environmental, socioeconomic, and personal lifestyle factors. It has been pointed out that those who become obese have reached that state of weight gain by the time they are in their mid-thirties, a decade or more younger than the age at which most of the long-term harmful health consequences of obesity begin. This reveals that, similar to other chronic diseases, such as heart disease and diabetes, obesity also has a long latency period between the exposure to risk factors and the onset of the condition, and once reached, its reversal is uncommon and is found in less than 15 percent of those who became obese in their mid-thirties.

Pre-Clinical Phase

Unlike other chronic diseases that may not manifest any outward symptoms at this stage, the appearance of obesity is both visible to the naked eye and measurable by determining the body mass index (BMI), a simple and cost-effective method. The presence of any associated, abnormal internal changes, however, would not be apparent, and would need to be assessed by diagnostic tests and clinical evaluation.

Clinical Phase

This begins when the disease is past its latency state and has entered the phase when one or more *co-morbidities* (e.g. type-2 diabetes, cardiovascular disease) may be manifested. Just as the cause of obesity involves many factors, its treatment is also based on multiple factors, including its severity and the presence of co-existing diseases.

It often involves a team approach, consisting of a physician, a registered dietician, and a psychologist or social worker; and a referral to a personal trainer or exercise physiologist may also be warranted. Bariatric surgery is only considered effective treatment in cases of severe or extreme obesity where significant, and sustained weight loss is desired, and only a small fraction of those eligible undergo this surgery. Not all physicians, including primary care physicians and those in subspecialties, are well equipped to manage the disease of obesity. Supported self-management, counseling for lifestyle changes, and referral to commercial weight-loss programs (those that successfully aid in sustainable weight loss and don't employ gimmicks) are strategies that have proven effective in treating obesity. Given the challenges involved in reversing obesity, prevention efforts should focus particularly on those who are just transitioning into adulthood and exhibit any level of being overweight.

Pathophysiology (abnormal physiological changes)

Pathophysiology involves any abnormal changes in the body, and this becomes clear as people approach the first visible stages of excess fat storage in the body that turns into overweight and obesity. It has long been known that people differ in terms of where they tend to store fat in the body. Men tend to store fat around their abdomen, which gives them that characteristic male pattern of fat distribution, or central obesity if they reach that level of body mass (BMI 30 or over). In women, fat tends to be stored more in their thighs and gluteal regions, the latter reflected in their having larger hip circumferences typical of the female pattern of fat distribution. Although abdominal fat storage is more common in men, it can also be seen in women, especially in the higher grades of obesity. Both in men and women, increased abdominal fat is associated with many co-existing diseases of obesity, including cardiovascular disease, and type-2 diabetes. Fat distribution is expressed by the waist-to-hip ratio (WHR), a measure regarded as critical in assessing the risks associated with obesity. It is derived by measuring the waist circumference at the natural waistline with a measuring tape, and dividing this by the hip circumference, measured at the maximal circumference of the hips, including the buttocks (e.g. 42"/44" yielding a WHR of 0.95). Men are considered at risk for obesity if the WHR is greater than 0.95, and a WHR greater than 0.80 puts women at risk for obesity.[23]

The size and number of fat cells are also recognized as being important in some complications associated with obesity, especially such metabolic disorders as glucose intolerance and type-2 diabetes. When obesity occurs during adult years or during pregnancy, it is mainly the result of an enlargement of fat cells, known as *hypertrophic* (a small number of large cells) obesity, and is more often associated with metabolic complications. But when the onset of obesity takes place in earlier years (childhood and adolescence), the fat cells turn over at a faster rate and multiply, resulting in a large number of smaller fat cells, and this type of obesity is known as *hyperplastic or hyper-cellular* (a large number of small cells) obesity. Nearly all those who reach or exceed a BMI of 35 (75 lbs. above normal body weight) have hyperplastic obesity, which is associated with an increase in triglyceride storage, and which, in turn, leads to an increased production of cholesterol and a decrease in high-density lipoprotein (HDL), the good cholesterol. These two factors account in part for the increased risk of cardiovascular diseases in the obese, but at any level of body fat, it is possible to have either type of obesity, regardless of the age or associated stage (such as pregnancy) of the onset of obesity.[24]

The association between obesity and a higher overall death rate, increased risk for heart disease, type-2 diabetes, and some cancers has been reported extensively in the medical literature. Compared to people in the normal weight range, the risk for these diseases among those in the obese category has been estimated to be as much as 2.8 times higher, depending on the level of obesity. Weight gain is associated with an increased demand for insulin from the pancreas, which over time leads to insulin resistance and type-2 diabetes, with their own risks for cardiovascular diseases, including hypertension, stroke, and coronary artery disease. Extreme weight gain, seen in severe obesity (BMI 40 and over) carries its own risks as well, such as sudden death, reported to be as much as 13 times higher than for people of normal weight. Hippocrates is said to have made a similar observation more than 2000 years ago, when such extreme weight gain would have been rare, and many epidemiologists have since reiterated it. Cardiomegaly (enlargement of the heart) and an associated dysfunction of the heart muscle are some of the consequences of extreme weight gain, and sleep apnea (intermittent and temporary cessation of breathing) is also common among the obese, particularly in those who are severely obese. In women, obesity is associated with *hirsutism,* a condition characterized by excessive hair growth in unusual places that is caused by increased androgens, and is resolved with weight loss. In men, severe obesity leads to a lower concentration of free testosterone. Due to the varied associated disease conditions, including some life-threatening ones, obesity, especially severe obesity, requires frequent hospitalizations, taking a toll on the individual and his or her family, as well as contributing to high healthcare costs.

Complications

Death is the ultimate complication of obesity, and each year more than 100,000 people die of obesity-related causes in the United States, with an estimated $150 billion spent in associated healthcare costs per year[25]. The most common complications of obesity are type-2 diabetes, heart disease, high blood pressure, hyperlipidemia (an increase in fats in the blood), sleep apnea, and osteoarthritis. Obesity also increases the risk for some cancers, including renal, breast, uterine, and colon cancer. Obese individuals are sometimes found to have psychosocial problems, and face discrimination at school and in the workplace. Childhood obesity is also reported to be associated with a distorted body image.

ERICK'S TRANSFORMATION FROM AN UNDERWEIGHT NEWBORN TO AN OBESE ADOLESCENT

Eric is a fourteen-year-old boy who has been my patient since his birth in 2000. As a matter of fact, I happened to deliver him, as obstetrics was a part of my practice at the time. He was delivered by normal vaginal delivery at 37 weeks gestation. His mother had no pre- or perinatal maternal complications. Eric weighed only 5 lbs. 1 oz at birth, which is well below the average birth weight in the U.S. He did gain weight during his first year, reaching the 25th percentile mark for his age in both height and weight by his 1st birthday. He remained at the 25th percentile level until he reached his third birthday. Eric received all the recommended childhood immunizations and was treated for some of the usual childhood illnesses. He also reached all the developmental milestones during his first three years. After that Eric started gaining weight at a rapid rate, and at age 4, he reached the 90th percentile mark in weight for his age. Eric's percentile weight gain on his growth chart was shared with his parents and they were counseled about his rapid weight gain and its ill effects, and advised to place controls on his eating. They complained that Eric does not stop eating even when admonished to not eat as much. Eric continued to gain excessive weight over the next several years.

By age eleven, Eric reached a height of 4' 11" and weighed 150 pounds, which placed him above the 95th percentile for his age and gender, putting him in the obese category. His Blood Pressure was pre-hypertensive at 124/74 mm Hg. Again, during his well child visits, I discussed with Erick's parents about his continued excess weight gain, and the only way to bring it under control would be to cut down on his eating, and increasing his physical activity. I suggested that they get him to participate in age-appropriate outdoor sports, limit his television watching, and time spent playing computer games that promote extended periods of sitting, and as well to limit his between-meal snacks and avoid offering him calorie-dense ones like potato chips, and candy.

By age 13, Eric grew to a height of 5'5" and weighed 207 pounds, and his blood pressure of 128/68 mm Hg. remained in the pre-hypertensive range. His physical examination revealed hyperpigmentation and thickening of the skin folds around his neck and his knees, a skin condition frequently associated with obesity, and adult-onset diabetes. I recommended blood studies that included his fasting blood glucose (FBG), cholesterol, and thyroid levels. With the exception of his cholesterol levels, which were slightly elevated, other test values were all within the normal range. I referred Eric for nutritional counseling, and advised the whole family to consider attending a weight loss program of their choice. Eric's parents, though not obese, are both overweight.

Two months later, I saw Eric for an ear infection, and treated him for it. During that visit, when I asked his parents if they were getting nutrition counseling for Eric as I had recommended, they said they had not yet done so, but would set that up soon. They had also not enrolled Eric or themselves in a weight-loss program. Since the parents had been monitoring their own blood pressure (BP) at home, they also started checking Eric's blood pressure from time to time. They reported to me on this particular occasion that his BP measurements ranged between 123–152 systolic and 76–97 diastolic. When I checked his BP, it was indeed 152/70 mm Hg. At this point, Eric weighed 210 pounds I had not yet detected any sense of alarm in Eric's parents about his steady weight gain. So, I sat with the two of them, without Eric being in the room, and explained the health risks associated with obesity, emphasizing diabetes and cardiovascular diseases in particular. I also pointed out there was a high probability for obese children to become obese adults. Then I also brought Eric into the room and impressed on all of them that Eric's weight reduction warranted a team effort between Eric, his family, and myself as their healthcare provider. The parents verbalized their agreement, with Eric also conveying his agreement with a nod. We made a plan to achieve our goal. I would make a referral to a weight reduction program that several of my patients had success in achieving sustained weight loss, and all three of them would enroll, so Eric would feel motivated and supported in achieving his goal. We set the goal for Eric to bring his weight down to 175 pounds, without exceeding a weight loss of one pound per week. I gave them a written referral, specifying in it the goal for Eric's weight reduction. The family was to follow up with me one month from that date.

At the follow-up visit one month later, the family reported that they all had enrolled in a weight reduction program, and Eric proudly announced that he lost six pounds, and now weighed 204 pounds. Eric was quite happy about his accomplishment, and seemed to have a new-found motivation to continue with the program. He even proceeded to tell me everything he had been learning from the nutritionist about what foods he should eat, and in what quantities. He also started riding a bicycle around the neighborhood. I complimented Eric and his parents on Eric's accomplishment. When Eric was seen three months later, he had only lost 2 additional pounds (not uncommon as weight loss is easier to achieve initially, and takes increasingly more effort to lose additional weight). Eric continues to struggle with his diet and exercise program, but remains motivated to lose weight and does not seem discouraged with his slower progress. Eric's weight reduction goal at this point in time is a work in progress for all of us on his team.

MARIA'S HEALTH PROBLEMS AND THE STRATEGY THAT HELPED DISMANTLE THEM

Maria is a 47-year-old, single woman who was first seen by me in my office a few years ago. She had been diagnosed with type-2 diabetes six years earlier, suffered from asthma, and hypothyroidism. She was taking two medications for her diabetes, a thyroid pill and a diuretic for leg swelling. She was also using an inhaler off and on for asthma attacks. Her old medical record revealed that Maria also had a history of depression, but was not being treated for it at the time. She worked as a muni bus driver. Maria is 5' 4" tall, and weighed 291 pounds, which placed her BMI at 50 (a BMI of 40 or greater is regarded extreme obesity). On the day of her visit with me, her blood pressure was 144/94 mm Hg. (desired level for someone with diabetes is 130/80 mmHg or less). Her physical examination was normal except for evidence of varicose veins on both legs, and mild edema (swelling) of her feet. We brought her adult immunizations up-to-date, and ordered several blood tests. The results of her blood tests showed nearly all of her values to be in the abnormal range. These included fasting blood glucose, total and component cholesterol levels, and triglycerides. The one exception to her abnormal cholesterol levels was her LDL cholesterol, which was well below 100 mg/dL, despite her not taking the cholesterol-lowering medication prescribed for her. Her thyroid hormone level was normal as well. A repeat measurement of her blood pressure showed it to be 140/90 mmHg. Based on these results, Maria met the criteria for, and was diagnosed with the following disease conditions: 1) Metabolic Syndrome; 2) Uncontrolled Type-2 Diabetes; 3) Uncontrolled Hypertension; and 4) Extreme Obesity. I explained to Maria, how each of these diseases affect her health individually and as co-existing conditions, and what lifestyle changes she needed to make, in addition to following prescribed treatment regimens.

I decided, in order for Maria to work actively to improve her physical health, her depression also needed to be addressed, and started her on treatment for depression. Maria responded well to her treatment, and her whole attitude toward her health improved greatly and she started taking more responsibility for her own health. Maria made some big changes in her diet and started exercising. She managed to lose 25 pounds on her own without the aid of any weight loss program. The modest weight loss (8.6%), coupled with some adjustments to her medications showed immediate and significant improvement in her blood chemistry values, bringing them to near normal levels across the board. If Maria continues on the current path, she will have her chronic health conditions under good control, and be able to manage her other health problems—asthma and hypothyroidism, and can look forward to a healthier future. Over the last three years that Maria has been under my care, she and I have been working diligently to reduce the severity of her obesity, and bring her diabetes and hypertension under better control.

The main take away from Maria's case is that when someone is suffering from depression, it can have a profound effect on all aspects of his or her life, including compliance with recommended actions for effective management of their physical health problems. Depression is a common, but a treatable disease, and it is critical to treat it concurrently with treatment of other co-existing health problems in order to achieve the optimum results, as was the case with Maria.

PART 3

Keeping Chronic Diseases at Bay or Stopping Them in Their Tracks

Part 3 addresses the right lifestyle choices to make and adhere to for life to prevent or forestall chronic diseases, as well as make their early detection and intervention possible when they do strike. In chapter 8, the desired lifestyle choices in seven key areas of daily living are described, along with multiple sources of available evidence that supports them. Regular and effective use of the recommended preventive health services is the subject of chapter 9. The economic and human costs of the major chronic diseases are addressed in the tenth and final chapter.

8

Making and Keeping the Right Lifestyle Choices

Lifestyle practices that have a strong impact on health are learned during the formative years and beyond, and usually begin in the home with parents or other adults. As social scientists tell us, health behavior is like any other human behavior, and once learned, a change in behavior, big or small, is daunting and can be stressful. Your eating habits, for example, are one such learned behavior, cultivated for the most part in childhood and continued into adulthood, until you are exposed to other practices you may adopt by choice or by necessity. This often happens when people move from one place to another, such as a different city or region within the same country, or an entirely different country. When exposed to new foods and new ways of eating them, you may slowly adopt these, especially if you are often eating in communal places. The same can also be true of other lifestyle practices, such as exercising, smoking, or drinking. Be aware that the habits in the place you migrated to may not always be better than those of the people you left behind, as in the following example. Many years ago, while I was attending graduate school in a college town, a fellow student from Sweden inquired of a local man where could he find good walking trails. Wanting to be helpful, the man asked him if he did not possess a car, because, he said, the roads in that town were excellent and he should be able to drive to anyplace he wanted to go and not have to walk. This misunderstanding completely defeated the purpose of the enquiry, of course, because the Swedish student wanted to walk for exercise.

After reading the topics covered in Parts 1 and 2, you may have inferred that the elements of lifestyle that have the highest impact on your health, especially with regard to chronic disease development, are the foods you eat (or don't eat) on a regular basis, the level of physical activity you engage in (from none to low, medium or high intensity), and whether or not you smoke tobacco and drink alcohol in excess (beyond moderation). If you did infer that, you would be right. However, there are other factors that contribute to, or deter you from achieving a healthy life, such as getting adequate rest and sleep, managing your stress effectively, maintaining meaningful personal relationships with others and having a strong support system.

MAKING YOUR EATING BOTH HEALTHFUL AND PLEASURABLE

You may be thinking that combining the two terms, *healthful* and *pleasurable,* in the context of eating is oxymoronic, but it is not because they need not be mutually exclusive. The perception that they are contradictory generally stems from two sources. First, from the often-conflicting stream of dietary advice dispensed through the sound bites of mass media about foods that are good or bad for you. Second, from the ubiquitous, much-ballyhooed commercial diet plans, mainly focused on weight loss (often-rapid), and make distinctions between good and bad foods strictly from the perspective of weight loss. The proponents of these diets aim for their customers to achieve the promised weight loss by restricting the kind of foods dieters eat, in some cases drastically. That, in fact, is the reason why, for many, the term 'diet' conjures up images of restricted eating for a limited duration for the sole purpose of losing weight. Used in this way, the term *diet* has essentially been hijacked by the commercial diet industry and deviates from its original meaning, which is to describe the foods a person or animal habitually eats. The dieting business has grown into a multi-billion-dollar industry, with promises of a specified amount of weight loss in a defined period, such as ". . . *help you lose 30 lbs. in six weeks."* There is a wide array of diets in the market with names and intriguing themes that most of us would not have heard of a few years ago. Many lack hard evidence that they are nutritionally sound or lead to sustained weight loss in the long run. A majority, if not all, of these diets are doomed to fail because they are inherently a short-term, Band-Aid solution to a longstanding problem. People who do manage to lose weight (often the ones giving the testimonials in TV commercials) on such diets usually gain it back (plus some), resulting in what has come to be known as yo-yo diets. The diet industry, however, keeps cashing in on this trend when the focus should instead be on healthy eating, with the goal of achieving and maintaining a healthy weight for the long run.

In doing research for this book, we encountered the statement "Americans are eating themselves to death" more than a few times, a reference to both the large portion size and poor nutritional quality. Overweight and obesity are health problems with potentially serious health consequences and, like any persistent health problems, warrant intervention by the combined efforts of trained professionals like nutritionists, registered dieticians, and physicians. If your weight is more than 10 percent above the ideal body weight for your height (two-thirds of the people in the U.S. are reported to be in this category), it is likely an indication of an energy imbalance (you are taking in more than you are expending). To achieve optimal weight loss in a healthy way, you would do well to be guided and monitored by health-care professionals who would help lead you to a healthy eating pattern, one that's not overly prescriptive or restrictive, but well-balanced and consistent with the broad principles and guidelines proven to be health-promoting and disease-preventing. Prevailing science supports a well-diversified diet slanted in favor of more plant-based foods, fewer animal products, and little to no processed foods. This is captured very succinctly by the best-selling author, Michael Pollan, in a single phrase on the cover of one of his books, *The Omnivore's Dilemma,* that reads, "Eat food. Not too much. Mostly plants."[1] To this, we would like to add our own earnest advice: enjoy what you eat and the eating itself, but do so in moderation. These two pieces of advice about eating can best be combined into one statement: Keep it small, sustainable, enjoyable, and diversified (KISSED, an easy-to-remember acronym). The key message here is, if you eat small portions of a broad variety of foods in an unhurried, relaxed manner that allows you to enjoy what you eat and the eating itself, over time you are likely to sustain that pattern of eating. One reason why most of the commercially available diets fail—and they do fail, or else there would not be the overweight and obesity problem there is today, considering the large percentage of people on some type of diet at any given time—is their lack of sustainability over a period of time. At best, they aid in a temporary weight loss. The diet is not sustainable in the long run because dieters tire of it, get discouraged and lose confidence by not achieving the results as fast as they expected, feel deprived by the restrictions, and may not enjoy the food they're allowed to eat, and sooner or later give up. Another reason for the failure is a built-in complexity, as most commercial diets require careful selection of foods by counting calories, making an evaluation of each food by its contribution to the proportion of recommended daily values, keeping a food journal, and possibly having to weigh the food, all of which make eating a chore and food seem more like medicine than pleasure. We firmly believe that, besides eating for nourishment, people eat food for pleasure, and this aspect of it should never be compromised. It is, in fact, critical for sustaining any eating pattern over the course of time.

Perhaps everyone could learn something from the French who are known to eat small helpings of a variety of foods and who enjoy every single morsel in an unhurried, relaxed manner. The French do not seem to have the problem of overweight and obesity to the extent that the U.S. has (overweight and obesity are four times more prevalent in the U.S. than in France), so the caveat here seems to be to eat a broad mix of foods in small quantities, and not eat at your desk or in the car. Instead, choose pleasant surroundings, and eat in the company of others whenever possible. Yes, the word *small* is relative, but suffice it to say that portions should be smaller than the ones two out of three Americans are likely eating now, and the amount that everyone in the U.S. used to eat before portions got supersized, thanks in part to the fast food chain restaurants.

A DIET TIP THAT WORKS

The co-author of this book, a practicing physician, has an interesting anecdote to share. After counseling his patients who needed to lose weight about cutting down on the size of their food portions and getting the same response from many of them, "But, doctor, I don't eat that much," he decided to try a different approach. He advised them to put the usual portions of food on their plate, but then remove a fifth (20 percent) of the food from each item on the plate, and eat only what remains. If they did not feel full afterward, he suggested they eat an apple or some other fruit.

Those who followed his recommendations reported being quite satisfied with the smaller portions (20 percent less food). Some even reported they had more energy after a reduced-portion meal because they didn't feel sluggish as they often had after a larger meal. More importantly, if they kept up with the slightly reduced portions, and added some regular moderate-intensity exercise, they lost weight and found it easier to maintain the weight loss for the long run, all this while enjoying the foods they liked, albeit in smaller quantities.

It's important to eat a variety of foods, and also to slant the mix in favor of more plant-based ones. The rationale for this recommendation is based on three facts.

- First, the current Western diet, particularly in the U.S., consists of meat and meat products in excess of the amount deemed healthy, due to their high saturated-fat content, and the insufficient amount of fiber in them, both of which are associated with an increased risk for chronic diseases like coronary artery disease and type 2 diabetes.

- Second, in addition to the vitamins and minerals the body needs, the plant-based foods contain phytochemicals (plant chemicals) that have health-promoting and disease-preventing properties (*lycopene* in tomatoes; *isoflavones* in soybeans, for example) that animal-based foods lack.

- Third, unlike animal-based foods, plant-based ones are not calo-rie-dense, and thus eating plant-based foods in larger volume (the only exception to the small-portion rule) helps a person reach satiety without contributing to a high calorie intake. As stated above, eating that is based on a rigid, restrictive, unbalanced approach, and focused primarily on weight loss, is not healthy eating. Much of the time, such a diet even fails to meet its intended goal of long-term weight loss.

Healthy eating should instead be guided by broad, proven, health and nutritional principles customized to individual circumstances because what people eat is driven largely by regional, cultural, and personal preferences. Above all, the reward from eating healthy has to be intrinsic, one that each person can feel good about and celebrate, and not just be about losing weight or coming down a dress size or two. If this all sounds a little too Pollyannaish, the elements of healthy eating are captured in the following eight broad principles.

Eight Key Elements of Healthy Eating

1. A healthy diet is balanced in the following approximate proportions of energy (measured in kilocalories) from macronutrients: 15 percent from proteins, 55 to 65 percent from carbohydrates, and 20 to 30 percent from fats. Both proteins and carbohydrates yield 4 kilocalories of energy per gram, while fats yield 9 kilocalories of energy per gram. The proportions should be used as an overarching principle for the total foods consumed in the course of the day and are not to be obsessed over at every single meal.

   - Proteins in the diet provide the amino acids necessary for the growth and repair of tissue, and can be obtained from a variety of plant and animal food sources, such as legumes, meats and poultry, seafood, and low-fat dairy products.

   - Carbohydrates are a basic source of energy for the body, to carry out both the internal metabolic functions and the external activities of daily living. They are stored in the body as glycogen, primarily in the liver and muscles as a source of reserve energy. The basic sources of carbohydrates are grains and starchy foods like potatoes. Whole grains are nutritionally superior to refined grains because the bulk of micronutrients (vitamins and minerals) are concentrated in the outer coats of the grain, which are largely removed in the process of refining. The Dietary Guidelines for Americans recommend that at least half the grains consumed be whole grains (e.g. whole wheat bread and pasta, brown rice, quinoa).

• Dietary fat supplies the body with the essential fatty acids needed for normal growth. Fats are stored as reserve energy in the form of triglycerides, to be used when needed, and they spare the proteins for other functions. In addition, subcutaneous fat provides some insulation to the body from heat loss, and cushions internal organs. Fats also serve as a medium for the fat-soluble vitamins A, D, E, and K that are needed for many vital body functions. However, not all fats are equally healthy and good for you. The mono- and polyunsaturated fats contained in olive oil and other vegetable oils are regarded healthy fats, while foods containing saturated fats, as in meats and full-fat dairy products, eaten in excess, are known to promote atherosclerosis (hardening of the arteries).

• Water is a critical nutrient, and has multiple roles in maintaining the homeostasis (equilibrium of the internal environment) of the human body. It achieves this by serving as a body's building base, solvent, reaction medium and reactant, carrier for nutrients and waste products, thermo regulator, lubricant, and shock absorber. A significant reduction in water intake can cause dehydration, and in severe form can (rarely) result in death. While healthy adults can withstand mild forms of dehydration without undue negative effects, young children and older people are less able to withstand its ill effects. The often-repeated admonition to drink at least eight 8-oz. glasses of water a day does not appear to have any scientific basis, nor can this advice be traced to any documented set of data. One researcher's quest to find out if there is indeed any scientific evidence to support drinking this huge amount of water turned out to be futile. Based on an extensive search of literature and discussions with nutritionists, this researcher suggests that the optimal fluid intake should be determined by individual physical and environmental conditions—body weight, physical activity, and the climate.[2] In studies carried out in Canada, the Netherlands, the United Kingdom, and the United States in the 1990s, the average daily per-capita water consumption was found to be less than 2 *liters* (eight glasses) with no negative effects. Given this ambiguity about the amount of water or total fluid intake in the course of a day, a sensible approach would be to drink water throughout the day, in amounts warranted by physical and environmental conditions, to maintain a healthy level of hydration.

2. A healthy diet is one that contains less of the animal-based foods and more of the plant-based ones. If you are a vegetarian or vegan, you can eat healthy on a diet based entirely on plant sources, but if you are a meat-eater, you should not eat a diet exclusively, or even predominantly, consisting of animal foods, as that can increase your risk for several chronic diseases. Instead, eat small amounts from leaner animals—lamb, turkey, chicken, and seafood—and eat meats from large animals (beef, pork) less often, preferably no more than two to three times a month. Fill three-quarters of your plate with plant-based foods—vegetables including green leafy ones, beans (or bean products like tofu), peas, lentils, fruits, nuts, and seeds. This will ensure that, in addition to getting your daily requirements of vitamins and minerals, you will also take in the recommended amount of fiber (25–30 grams)—Americans take in only half that amount on average.

   • Fiber, also known as roughage, is not really a nutrient, and is not digested or absorbed by the body, but it is nevertheless a much-needed component of your diet. There are two kinds of fiber, soluble and insoluble, that perform different, important functions. The soluble fiber, so called because it is soluble in water, forms a gel-like substance in the digestive tract, and acts as a scavenger by binding to particles of LDL cholesterol (the bad kind) and preventing it from entering the bloodstream. Both soluble and insoluble fiber help in slowing the emptying of food from the stomach, thereby delaying absorption of the sugar in the food. By maintaining satiety longer, this keeps hunger in check between meals, and prevents a sudden rise and fall in blood-glucose levels, an important benefit for everyone, but especially for those with type-2 diabetes or pre-diabetes. The insoluble fiber also provides the bulk needed to regularly move the bowels. With the triple duty fiber does, it is clearly beneficial, and indispensable to your health, and a minimum of 25 grams (30 grams is desirable) should be part of the daily diet. Fiber is found only in plants, therefore only in plant-based foods—fruits, vegetables (including root and leafy vegetables), and whole grains.

- Super foods is a label reserved for foods known to be superior for contributing to health and longevity, and 80–90 percent of these come from such plant-based foods as almonds, apples, beans, most berries, oats, mushrooms, pomegranate, pumpkin, spinach, and tea. Therefore, if you eat more plant-based foods, there is a greater likelihood of your getting more super foods into your diet, a simple but true and powerful fact.

- Generally, the richest sources of vitamins, minerals, and the much-touted antioxidants, as well as fiber, are the dark green, yellow and orange-colored vegetables and fruits, the green leafy vegetables (such as kale, spinach, chard), carrots, pumpkin, yams, red, orange, and yellow bell peppers, apples, oranges, papayas, mangos, and berries (most kinds, but the darker the color the more nutrient-rich they are, like the blue and black berries).

3. Limit sugar and added salt intake.

- The American Heart Association recommends that women consume no more than the equivalent of 6 teaspoons of sugar per day, and men no more than 9 teaspoons. This includes sweeteners you use in your coffee, tea, or other beverages. Sugar in any form is known to promote inflammation in the body, which, in turn, leads to cellular damage and aging, so limiting your sugar intake helps to slow down the aging of cells. This does not mean total abstinence from your favorite dessert, only that you should limit it in portion size and frequency.

- Most foods naturally contain sodium in varying amounts. Added salt (sodium chloride or table salt) should be limited to 1500–2000 mg (about a tea spoon) per day, the less the better. Try substituting herbs and spices (without added salt) for salt to enhance the taste and flavor of food. There are many wonderful herbs (e.g. basil, mint, oregano, rosemary, thyme) and spices available on the market, both locally grown and imported, and in addition to being taste and flavor boosters, some, like cumin, ginger, and turmeric, have other known health benefits.

4. Fat is not your enemy, but if you take in too much of the wrong kind, it can work against you. You do need some dietary fat, but it's important to be selective in the kinds of fats you consume—mono-unsaturated fats vs. saturated fats for example. As a rule of thumb, eat more unsaturated fats, restrict saturated fats, and avoid trans fats in order to optimize the health-protective benefits of fat, and minimize its negative effects. The sources of the unsaturated fats are vegetable oils—olive oil, canola oil, nut, and seed oil, nut but-ters (e.g. almond butter), and avocado. Saturated fats are found in butter, margarine, and all meats and full-fat dairy products. Hydro-genated oils like shortening contain trans fats that are best avoided. Be aware that manufacturers are legally allowed to list foods with 0.5 grams or less trans fats per serving as containing *zero trans fats* on the nutrition label.

5. Do not skip breakfast, an admonishment you have probably heard ad nauseam. So what is behind it? Science, actually, with study after study correlating the regular eating of breakfast with better health, and skipping it with poorer health. There's a reason why the first meal of the day is called breakfast (or break-the-fast) as it literally means stopping the fast since the last meal of the prior night. Your

blood sugar is at its lowest level when you wake up because no food was taken in during the night to stimulate glucose production. This is why, when your doctor orders a fasting blood-sugar test, you are asked not to eat or drink for at least eight hours prior to the test. That age-old saying to eat breakfast like a king, lunch like a prince, and dinner like a pauper, is sage advice in principle. This pattern of eating ensures that you are front-loading your calories for energy expenditure throughout the day, and taking in fewer calories at the back end when energy demands are likely to be lower.

6. Eat small portions. Granted the term *small* is relative, but it is now recognized as a fact that eating larger portions of food is one of the major factors contributing to the unprecedented rise in overweight and obesity rates in the U.S. One example of how supersized portions are made more alluring is the common gimmick that fast food restaurants use of selling double servings, (e.g. two burgers) for the price of one, or selling the second burger for a minimal additional price. This helps them increase their sales and profits, as the additional food does not entail additional fixed costs for the restaurant. The phrase *supersizing America* has been coined to capture this trend of larger servings, both at home and when eating out. The excess food consumed, however, is stored as fat in the body, which is reflected in the unprecedented rise of overweight and obesity, and the associated increase in several chronic diseases, as described.

7. When eating between meals (most people do), replace calorie-dense and nutrition-poor foods like chips and sugary drinks with nutritious snacks like fruits and nuts. Snacks count in total calories consumed, so it is sensible to make them count for their nutritional value as well by snacking on nuts (almonds, walnuts, unsalted peanuts), seeds (pumpkin seeds, sunflower seeds), fruits, and raw vegetables.

8. Limit your alcohol intake. Science supports drinking in moderation (no more than one drink a day for women and two for men) as that has been associated with health benefits. Drinking small amounts of wine with food is an element of the much-touted Mediterranean

diet. But the caveat here is to drink in moderation because more of a good thing is certainly not better—excess alcohol consumption is not only hazardous to your health, but it can also endanger the health and safety of others due to actions taken by you while under the influence.

The essence of the key elements of healthy eating outlined above is also embedded in the Mediterranean diet, which has withstood the test of time. In a joint study by the University of Athens Medical School and The Harvard University School of Public Health, researchers sought to find out if adherence to the Mediterranean diet improved total mortality as well as mortality from coronary heart disease and cancer. The results, published in *The New England Journal of Medicine*, revealed the striking findings that this was indeed true.[3] Adherence to a traditional Mediterranean diet *was* inversely related to both total mortality and mortality from coronary heart disease and cancer. Even a partial adherence to the Mediterranean diet was associated with a marked reduction in mortality. The closer the adherence to the diet, the better the outcome (a reduction in death rate). In medical parlance, this incremental association between cause and effect is known as a *dose-response* relationship, and is indicative of the strength of the association between two factors. After remaining dormant in the last decades of the twentieth century, there seems to be a renewed interest in the Mediterranean diet worldwide, but the U.S. in particular, due to the burgeoning twin problems of overweight/obesity and the associated chronic diseases.

The Dietary Guidelines for Americans are jointly issued, and updated every five years, by the Department of Agriculture (USDA) and the Department of Health and Human Services (HHS). These guidelines are formulated by panels of experts from the fields of nutrition and health, and provide evidence-based, authoritative advice on healthy diet for Americans from age two and up. They are intended to help consumers make informed food choices for healthy eating, and coupled with the appropriate physical activity, are intended to help attain and maintain a healthy weight and reduce the risk for chronic diseases. The guidelines are made available to the public, healthcare institutions, and nutrition and health professionals in a variety of forms, including a dedicated website, ChooseMyPlate.gov (formerly MyPyramid.gov), and printed materials provided on request. The website, which provides a wealth of information to consumers on a range of nutrition-related topics, is presented in a user-friendly and instructive manner with attractive visuals. While there is a tendency for some to be skeptical about any information, health information in particular, provided by a governmental agency like the USDA, we found the information on the website to be current, comprehensive, and evidence-based. The food pyramid, used for decades by USDA to illustrate the relative amounts of the different nutrients to be included in the daily diet, has been replaced by 'My Plate', an image depicting a dinner plate, divided into four unequal sections, each filled with a food group. In the image, three-quarters of the plate is filled with plant-based foods (half the plate with fruits and vegetables, and one quarter with grains), and the remaining space is reserved for protein-rich foods like meats, beans, and nuts. We took an in-depth look at these guidelines to determine if what we outlined in the eight key elements of healthy eating is consistent with the current USDA guidelines and concluded that the two are consistent, both substantively and in the broader principles.

Be Smart about Food Shopping

Healthy eating begins with choices made while shopping for food, whether it is at a supermarket, a farmers' market, or a bulk store. Smart, informed choices made while food shopping lead to healthy eating, and poor choices result in the opposite. Many people invest more time and thought into buying other things than into buying food to eat, even though the latter is far more intimately connected with health and wellbeing. Even the time of the day chosen to do food shopping can influence choices in grocery aisles. If you stop by the store on your way home from work and are in a rush to get home and prepare dinner, help the kids with homework, or attend to any number of other tasks, you're not likely to invest much time weighing your choices and choosing the best option. Consequently, the subliminal messages of the advertisers or the artful displays of the grocer could dictate your choices, none of which may necessarily turn out to be the healthiest. Similarly, shopping while hungry may tempt you to buy prepared foods that are ready to eat, which again may not be as healthy a choice as you would otherwise make. Simply making a shopping list in advance, writing down specific items along with brand names and quantities desired, can help minimize making wrong food choices.

Get to know the food you are buying. If it's a fruit or vegetable item, learn if it is grown locally, trucked in from clear across the country, or imported from another country. If locally grown, it's likely to have been freshly harvested before being brought to the market and hasn't been in transport for days or weeks. Local fruits and vegetables would have been allowed to grow until they reached their peak nutritional quality, instead of being harvested prematurely to allow for a lengthy transport.

When buying a non-produce item, read the nutritional label and the list of ingredients on the package. The Nutrition Labeling and Education Act of 1990 mandated that standardized nutrition information appear on almost all packaged foods manufactured after 1994. Reading and understanding nutrition labels on foods may be an important step toward healthy eating, and for this reason consumers are increasingly being advised to read nutrition labels before selecting their purchase. There have been systematic attempts to study how consumers use nutrition labels and what effect reading labels has on dietary behaviors, and findings consistently point to a relationship between consumers reading the labels and their dietary practices. One study conducted with adults from four family-medicine clinics in Southeastern Missouri revealed that those test subjects who ate diets lower in fat and higher in fruits, vegetables, and fiber reported that label reading had had an influence on their food-purchase decisions. This occurred with them much more frequently than with those test subjects whose diets were higher in fat (51 percent versus 26 percent).[4] In this study, those with high blood pressure were 63 percent more likely to look for sodium content on the nutrition label than those with normal or low blood pressure. And those with high cholesterol were more likely to look for saturated fat on the label than those with normal or low cholesterol. The data on label reading show that the practice is associated with a lower intake of fat; it is significantly higher among women, people younger than thirty-five years of age, and those with more than a high school education. The strongest predictors of label use, however, were a belief in the importance of eating a low-fat diet, being in the process of adopting a low-fat diet, or believing in the association between diet and cancer. Label use was not associated with the consumption of fruits and vegetables in this study.

There are a few key factors to look for when reading nutrition labels. The first one is the serving size, as all other numbers on the label are listed per serving. Determining the exact serving size may require simple arithmetic as the label often lists only the total number of servings. A serving size is simply the quantity derived by dividing the total content amount of the package by the number of servings (e.g. the serving size in a 16-oz. package meant for four servings is 16/4 = 4 oz.). The other key factors to read include the total calories and calories from fat, the amount of saturated and trans fats, and fiber. If a serving of a food contributes more than 25 percent of its calories from fat, the food is regarded a high-fat food, and needs to be balanced with a lower-fat food in the same, or another, meal, preferably in the same day. Generally accepted dietary guidelines recommend limiting the intake of saturated fat to less than 7 percent of total energy, trans fat to less than 1 percent of energy (if a food contains less than 0.5 grams of trans fat, manufacturers are allowed to list it as containing zero trans fat), dietary cholesterol to less than 300 mg per day, sodium not to exceed 2300 mg per day, and a minimum of 25 grams of fiber a day. To date, available data point to the fact that people who successfully limit their fat intake use nutrition labels, suggesting that reading the nutrition labels is useful in this regard. However, not everyone may find the nutrition labeling entirely reader-friendly. Dieticians often offer help, upon request, in the correct reading and interpretation of the various numbers listed on the nutrition labels, some even leading groups in grocery stores, to teach how to use nutrition labels to make healthy food purchases. If you're buying packaged or processed foods (keep these to a minimum, or preferably avoid them altogether), read those labels for nutritional content, as well as for additives and pre-servatives. If an item is imported from another country, their package and nutrition labeling may be different from the U.S. standard and may warrant additional scrutiny.

Increasingly, another dilemma being faced by consumers in food shopping is whether or not to buy organic, and what foods, if any, would be worth paying the extra money for. The term "organic" means food produced in a way that complies with standards set by national governments and international organizations. In the United States, organic food production is a system managed in accordance with the Organic Foods Production Act (OFPA) of 1990, and regulations in Title VII. The USDA carries out routine inspections of farms that produce USDA Organic-labeled foods. The possible adverse health effects of foods produced using intensive farming methods has led to concerns among consumers, and has given rise to considerable interest in organically produced crops and animal products. Some even refer to the slow, but steady rise in organic farming as the *organic food movement*. Organic farming uses no synthetic (chemical) pesticides or fertilizers to produce food, although certain organically approved pesticides may be used under limited conditions. In general, organic foods are not processed using irradiation, industrial solvents, or chemical food additives, and are often processed with fewer artificial methods, such as chemical ripening and genetically modified ingredients. In the case of organic meat production, the livestock are reared free-range with regular access to a pasture, and without the routine use of antibiotics or growth hormones. Organic meat certification in the United States authenticates that the farm animal products meet USDA organic food protocol, e.g., organic meats, poultry, and dairy products come from animals raised *free-range* instead of in the feedlots. Seafood is considered the equivalent of organic if it is wild-caught, instead of farm-raised in artificial and crowded conditions. Foods sold as organic require producers to obtain special certification based on government-defined standards in order to market any food as organic. There is a widespread perception among consumers that such (organic) methods of food cultivation result in foods of higher nutritional quality. A limited number of studies have compared the nutrient compositions of organically and conventionally produced crops, and an even smaller number of studies comparing meats and dairy products produced under free-range and conventional systems. The small and inconsistent differences found in these studies led to the conclusion that between the two types of food, there probably are no nutritionally important differences in the contents of minerals, vitamins, proteins, and carbohydrates. This is bolstered by the fact that typical first-world diets are not deficient in these nutrients, and the levels of pesticide residues in conventional products are not a cause for concern. The same studies, however, did consistently find higher nitrate (used as fertilizer) and lower vitamin-C contents in conventionally produced vegetables, particularly leafy vegetables. This finding might constitute a case for buying organic vegetables, leafy ones in particular. The authors of one particular study recommended more and better research than is currently available in order to validate (or refute) consumer perceptions regarding the potential health benefits of organic foods.[5]

Although health and food-safety concerns are the main motives for organic food purchases, for many, ethical concerns, particularly in relation to animal welfare, also play a significant role in the decision to purchase organic food. Such ethical considerations drive the purchase of organic food and free-range products, and can therefore be viewed as interrelated because the buyers of such products also associate them with higher standards of food safety and healthfulness. There is no scientific evidence to date of any benefit or harm to human health from a diet high in organic food, and no long-term studies have been done on the health outcomes of populations consuming predominantly organic versus conventionally produced food. The prevailing evidence for the health benefits of organic foods does not support a blanket recommendation for buying organic, either selectively or in entirety. The current market share of organic foods is quite small, ranging between 3–5 percent, and the consumers of organic foods are not homogeneous in demographics or in their beliefs about the benefits of organically cultivated foods. Women, and those under the age of thirty-five, are reported to dominate the regular buyers of organic food. At first, many associate organic with vegetables and fruits, and their organic purchases start with them, then progress to other organic products, such as meats and dairy, while some continue to limit their organic buying to fruits and vegetables.

Be Physically Active

Health benefits can be derived from moderate-intensity exercise. Your weight is a reflection of energy intake and energy output. If you take in more than you expend, the excess gets stored as fat in the body and results in weight gain. If you take in less energy than you expend, you will lose weight over a period of time. The second most important component of the two-part equation (the first is diet, detailed above) is your level of physical activity. It determines whether you maintain a healthy weight or become overweight or obese and risk the consequences of ill health. It has long been recognized that the levels of physical activity and physical fitness significantly influence the risk for chronic disease and premature death, and a mountain of data that confirms this has been generated. How much and what level of physical activity is necessary to stay healthy and lower the risk of chronic disease is a question asked by researchers studying the association between physical activity and disease and death rates from all causes, and from chronic diseases, cardiovascular diseases and diabetes in particular.

The summary findings of several credible studies on this topic are presented here.

A Study of Harvard University Male Alumni

The study was conducted to examine the association between exercise habits and deaths from all causes and from coronary heart disease among the male alumni of Harvard University over a ten-year period.[6] This study revealed that, even when taken up later in life, participating in regular physical activity of at least moderate intensity, quitting cigarette smoking, maintaining normal blood pressure, and avoiding overweight and obesity were each individually, and collectively, associated with lower rates of death from all causes as well as from coronary heart disease. These findings endured over time as was shown by their consistency from two measurements taken ten years apart. The association also persisted across age groups, indicating that lifestyle practices of being sedentary, smoking cigarettes, being overweight (for height), and having high blood pressure each carried with it a higher risk for disease, and premature death regardless of age.

Over all, the sedentary men showed a 25-percent higher risk of death than the more active men, and those men who did not engage in any sports activity that was at least moderately vigorous had a 44-percent higher risk of death than those who did engage in such activity. The group that engaged in moderately vigorous sports activity also had a 41-percent lower risk of dying from coronary heart disease. Finally, this study examined the effects of lifestyle changes and adoption of low-risk practices on longevity, even when these were made in mid-life. On average, taking up moderately vigorous sports activity added seven tenths of a year (0.72), and giving up smoking added one and one half (1.46) years, but doing both gained them an extension of two and one half (2.49) years of life on average. In this study, there were two noteworthy findings with respect to physical activity. One was that any level of physical activity has health benefits, with an incremental rise in benefits with greater intensity and longer duration of activity, and the second was that the benefits are compounded when combined with giving up an unhealthy practice like smoking.

The evidence that moderate-intensity activity is associated with a reduction in the risk of coronary heart disease has been mounting for decades. More than forty epidemiologic studies have addressed the relation between exercise and heart disease. The risk reduction is reported to be between 30–50 percent in both men and women who engage in regular physical activity.

The Nurses' Health Study, 1986–1996

This large prospective study was done to determine the effects of walking versus vigorous exercise in preventing coronary heart disease in women.[7] In 1986, more than 72,000 female nurses between the ages of forty and sixty-five years participated in the study. For each of the participants, the average amount of time spent per week during the previous year, in the following activities was recorded:

- Walking or hiking outdoors, such as walking to work or while playing golf;

- Jogging at a speed slower than ten minutes per mile;

- Running at ten minutes per mile or faster;

- Bicycling, including the use of a stationary bicycle;

- Swimming laps;

- Playing tennis or squash;

- Participating in calisthenics, aerobics, or aerobic dance;

- The average number of flights of stairs they climbed each week.

The women also reported their usual walking pace: easy or casual (from less than 2–2.9 mph), brisk (between 3.0–3.9 mph), or very brisk (4.0 mph or faster). The cumulative average number of hours per week spent in moderate or vigorous recreational activities (except for walking at a casual or average pace) was computed. The number of hours per week of moderate or vigorous activity was found to be strongly, and inversely (the greater the amount of time spent, the lower the risk) related to the risk of coronary events. Those who spent an average of 4.0–6.9 hours per week in moderate or vigorous recreational activities had a risk reduction of 31 percent, and the ones who spent an average of 7.0 or more hours per week in such activities experienced a 37 percent reduction in risk, compared with those who spent less than 1 hour per week on average in such activities. This clear incremental effect attests to the strong association between physical activity and the risk for heart disease. Women who were more physically active were also less likely to be current smokers and, as expected, they were leaner and had a lower prevalence of hypertension, diabetes, and hypercholesterolemia (high levels of cholesterol in blood) than less active women. Women who were more physically active were also more likely to use postmenopausal hormone-replacement therapy, nutritional supplements, and consume alcohol in moderation. During the follow-up period, there were 645 coronary events (475 nonfatal myocardial infarctions and 170 deaths from coronary disease) among the 72,488 women who were between forty and sixty-five-years of age in 1986, and did not have a history of heart disease. The total physical-activity score was strongly and inversely related to the risk of coronary events during the eight-year follow-up. The relationship was inverse and incremental; revealing that the higher the activity scores, the lower the risk of any coronary event. The level of activity was not related to age, smoking status, family history of myocardial infarction, or dietary intake of fats or cholesterol. Even after adjusting (removing the effects) for these factors, the total physical-activity score remained a powerful predictor of the subsequent risk of a coronary event. The relative risk for a coronary event among the lowest, and the highest activity scores ranged between 0.88 and 0.66. Stated another way, compared to the average risk of coronary event among the sedentary individuals, the risk among those who were active was 12 to 34 percent lower, the higher level of activity being associated with a larger decrease in risk. The walking pace was also an important determinant of the risk of coronary events, and it emerged as an independent predictor of the risk of coronary events. Compared with women who walked at an easy or casual pace, women who usually walked at an average pace (2.0–2.9 mph) had a relative risk of 0.75, whereas those who walked briskly or very briskly (above 3.0 mph) had a relative risk of 0.64. Women who engaged in both walking and vigorous exercise had greater reductions in coronary events than those who participated in either type of activity alone. In this study, the researchers pointed out that they did not find a greater risk reduction with vigorous exercise than with walking, as the degree of risk reduction associated with brisk walking and vigorous exercise were similar when total energy expenditures were similar. The findings of this prospective study indicate that both brisk walking and vigorous exercise are associated with substantial reductions in the incidence of coronary events. These findings lend further support to current exercise guidelines provided by The Centers for Disease Control and Prevention (CDC), which endorse moderate-intensity exercise for at least thirty minutes on most (preferably all) days of the week. Based on the results of their study, the researchers concluded that an exercise regimen, such as brisk walking for three or more hours per week, could reduce the risk of coronary events in women by 30–40 percent, and that increasing walking time or combining walking with vigorous exercise may yield even greater risk reductions. The researchers also estimated that one third of coronary events among middle-aged women in the United States are attributable to a lack of sufficient physical activity.

The Iowa Women's Health Study, 1986–2007

Another major study, investigated the association between physical activity and all-cause mortality in post-menopausal women. The findings revealed that both moderate activity and vigorous activity to be inversely related to overall mortality, and mortality due to cardiovascular causes. In both cases the relationship was incremental.[8] These findings also lend support to the current guidelines that endorse moderate-intensity exercise, which is safe, achievable, and feasible for the majority of the population. Findings from the studies cited here, as well as several others, support the inference that there is a causal link between regular physical activity of moderate intensity and a reduced risk of coronary events, such as a heart attack, and that the risk may be further reduced through vigorous activity, even when it is begun in later adulthood.

In order to derive health benefits for the long term, exercising, like healthy eating, should also be kept simple, enjoyable, diversified, and sustainable. Unlike incidental physical activity, purposeful exercising does require carving out time in the day, several times a week. Much like fad diets, getting on the bandwagon with the latest aerobic dance workout, or joining the gym because everyone you know is doing it may or may not work for you. Such activities often require driving to the venue, which takes up additional time above and beyond what is required by the activity itself. Picking an activity you can do only on weekends is not sufficient, as it would mean doing it only once or twice a week.

Traditionally, physical-activity recommendations have focused on the frequency, intensity, duration, and mode of the activity, like thirty minutes of moderate-intensity activity, such as brisk walking, on most days of the week. As the most commonly reported physical activity is walking, pedometers (worn on your clothing) provide a simple, practical, reliable, and affordable means of tracking the activity, expressed as a summary output of steps per day. *The 10,000 steps a day slogan,* associated with a healthful level of physical activity, can be traced to Japanese walking clubs in the 1960s when they began using the pedometer.[9] They nicknamed the pedometer in Japanese as *manpokei,* the literal translation being "the ten thousand steps meter." A study of the typical steps per day for various lifestyles in Japan established that, for an average middle-aged Japanese man, 10,000 steps translated to approximately 300 kcal burned. The concept of 10,000 steps a day, and the use of a pedometer to track them gained popularity not only in Japan, but in other parts of the world as well, including in the U.S. Ten thousand steps a day is a reasonable estimate of daily activity for healthy adults. Results from some studies suggest that a goal of 10,000 steps a day may not be sustainable for some groups, including older adults and those living with chronic diseases, and is probably too low for children, an important target population to prevent obesity. Pedometer-determined physical activity in healthy adults has been indexed as below.

- Less than 5,000 steps/day: Sedentary lifestyle;

- 5,000–7,499 steps a day: Low active (typical of daily activity, excluding sports/exercise);

- 7,500–9,999 steps: Somewhat active (likely includes some intentional physical activities or occupation-related physical tasks).

- 10,000–12, 499 steps/day: Active (level of physical activity recommended for optimal health benefits).

- 12,500 or more steps a day: High active (level of activity achieved by athletes in training, joggers, and runners).

With the exception of the last category, pedometer-determined physical activity can be achieved in increments, such as a ten-minute walk three times a day or a fifteen-minute walk twice a day, to more easily plug it into your daily schedule. Public health guidelines promote thirty minutes a day of moderate-intensity activity for adults. In walking for exercise, 100 steps a minute are said to be the minimal pace for moderate-intensity activity.

This last section has probably sparked a question as to whether exercise needs to be an intentional daily activity performed during a special time in order to gain the health benefits, or if it can be achieved through incidental daily activities like walking the dog, walking the children to school, climbing the steps instead of taking the elevator, parking farther and walking the distance, etc. Several years ago, I found the following sign posted by an elevator at a hospital, of all places, that stayed with me for its implied message. The elevator was in an area of the hospital that was used primarily by hospital staff, and the posted sign read as follows: *Climbing the stairs, instead of taking the elevator, is good for your heart. Taking the elevator to go down is simply a waste of electricity.* It was a small sign with a big message—move your body on your own as much as possible, rather than rely on a passive mode of transport. I believe the message on the sign also spoke to the desirability of incorporating incidental bouts of exercise into your daily life. At work and at home, if you seize every opportunity in the course of a day to move your body instead of remaining sedentary, your body will respond by remaining fit and healthy, and it will have the added benefit of helping you look trim.

Avoid Cigarette Smoking

Cigarette smoking continues to be one of the leading preventable causes of disease, disability, and death in the U.S. In the last half-century, there has been a great deal of research on the harmful effects of smoking on health.[10] According to the Centers for Disease Control and Prevention, in addition to diseases known to be caused by, or associated with, smoking, including bladder, esophageal, laryngeal, lung, oral, and throat cancers, new ones have been added to this list. These include an abdominal aortic aneurysm, acute myeloid leukemia, cataracts, and cervical cancer. Smoking is also recognized as a risk factor for infertility, preterm delivery, stillbirth, and sudden infant death syndrome (SIDS). Postmenopausal women who smoke have lower bone density, and an increased risk for hip fracture, than those who never smoked.[11] If you are a current smoker, it would be to your advantage to enroll in a program designed to help people stop smoking.

A group of researchers studied the effects of smoking cessation on longevity by determining, at various ages, how long life got extended when the person stopped smoking. They used a subset of participants in the Cancer Prevention Study II, an ongoing study of a cohort of 1.2 million U.S. adults that was begun in 1982.[12] From 1982 through 1996, after adjusting for such factors as alcohol intake, marital status, and education, they examined 877,000 respondents to determine the association between smoking and mortality. The researchers identified 149,351 deaths from all causes and they estimated mortality due to smoking by calculating the relative risk of death from all causes, stratified by age, race, sex, and smoking-status. Male smokers who quit at age thirty-five lived between 6.9–8.5 years longer than men who continued to smoke, and the corresponding increase in longevity among women ranged between 6.1–7.7 years. As expected, smokers who quit at younger ages (presumably shortening the duration of smoking) lived longer, but even those who quit much later in life gained some benefits. Among smokers who quit at age sixty-five, the men gained 1.4–2.0 years of life, and women gained 2.7–3.7 years. This relationship between the age at which a person stopped smoking and how long he/she lived reflects how powerful the association between smoking and longevity is. It also points out the importance of stopping smoking at any age for a meaningful extension of life, but the earlier a person stops smoking, the greater the longevity benefit.

One study estimated the expected lifetime economic consequences of cigarette smoking for individual smokers. These were arrived at by combining costs of three smoking-related diseases (lung cancer, coronary heart disease, and emphysema) with estimates of smokers' increased likelihood (specific to age and gender) of developing these illnesses in each remaining year of life, relative to nonsmokers. Both the economic costs of smoking and the benefits of quitting were calculated separately for men and women ages thirty-five to seventy-nine years who were light, moderate, or heavy cigarette smokers. The economic costs of smoking were significant for all groups of smokers, but varied by sex, age, and the amount smoked. For example, the lifetime costs for a forty-year-old man ranged from $20,000 for a smoker of less than one pack of cigarettes per day to over $56,000 for a smoker of more than two packs of cigarettes per day. The economic benefits of quitting smoking were also sizable for all groups of smokers. Some employers have started a system of providing incentives and disincentives to discourage their employees from smoking by giving rewards to those who smoke for quitting or participating in a smoking-cessation program, and penalties to those who continue to smoke. In motivating smokers to quit, the penalty-based incentives, such as a higher shared cost for health insurance, are reported to have generated more resistance than the reward-based incentives.[13]

Smoking rates have been declining in the last decade, and there has been a related increase in the number of cities and communities who have smoke-free laws to protect people living in those areas from toxic secondhand smoke in public places. There is also a growing societal pressure to stop smoking, including public service announcements and advertisements in mass media about smoking-related illnesses and their effect on individuals and their loved ones. However, one in six adults in the U.S. still smokes, and thousands die every year from a smoking-related illness. From a public health perspective, healthcare providers are primary, as they begin the systematic identification of smokers and supply a formal diagnosis of nicotine dependence.

Habitual smoking is an addiction, caused by the chemical nicotine in tobacco. Addiction of any kind is also a behavior, and overcoming it poses many challenges for the person and his or her loved ones. Social scientists who have studied the phenomenon of addiction and a person's ability to overcome it have explained it in terms of behavioral theories, such as the social cognitive theory, and the trans-theoretical model. The premise of social cognitive theory is that people learn by observing others, and imitate what they observe. A person may initiate smoking due to parental or other adult influence, but other environmental cues help maintain the behavior.[14] The trans-theoretical model is based on change of behavior that allows the person to develop strategies to change or modify a problem behavior or adopt a new positive behavior through four stages of change—pre-contemplation, contemplation, planning, and action.[15] Some have added maintenance and termination to these stages in order to fully address the gamut of behaviors needed for a successful change. This model of behavior modification has been successfully used in health education to determine if individuals are ready to change a problem behavior. Behavioral therapy alone has been successful in approximately 20 percent of smokers willing to participate.

The key components of an effective behavioral program are:

- An assessment of a smoker's readiness in terms of what stage of change he/she is in;

- Prompting the smoker to identify the perceived barriers to quitting;

- Development of plans for preventing a relapse.

Most smoking-cessation programs now combine behavioral therapy with drug therapy for higher rates of success.

Pharmacological (drug-based) Approaches to Smoking Cessation

For a majority of smokers wanting to quit, assistance with drug therapy, alone or in combination with other forms of therapy, remains the most attractive method to stop smoking. For many years, nicotine itself, the addictive chemical in tobacco, has been used in a therapeutic form to help a person stop smoking, and has, in fact, become the pharmacologic mainstay in this endeavor. The standard approach has been nicotine substitution, using one of the four forms of nicotine replacement currently available—gum, patch, nasal spray, and inhaler. The efficacy of each nicotine-replacement product is similar in achieving the cessation rate. Which form of nicotine delivery to use depends on individual preference, and should be decided on in consultation with a healthcare provider.

The nicotine patch. Nicotine in the form of a patch has been used as a therapeutic aid in smoking cessation for many years. A meta-analysis (of similar pooled studies) done to determine the overall efficacy of the nicotine patch for treating tobacco dependence revealed some significant findings. To avoid any bias in assessing results, it included seventeen double-blind nicotine-patch studies of four weeks or longer, (neither the participant nor the researcher knew who was receiving the drug nicotine, and who was getting the placebo), with laboratory confirmation of abstinence from tobacco, and a six-month follow-up after the treatment was completed. There were more than 5,000 participants in the pooled studies, and at the end of the treatment, the tobacco-abstinence rates for the nicotine patch vs. the placebo were 27 and 13 percent respectively, which indicated a two-times greater abstinence with the nicotine patch, compared to the placebo. Six months later, at 22 and 9 percent respectively, the corresponding proportions were even better. Regardless of the patch type (sixteen-hour or twenty-four-hour), duration of treatment, weaning, or the accompanying format or intensity of counseling, the nicotine patch proved superior to the placebo in maintaining abstinence from smoking. The intensive behavioral counseling had a reliable but modest positive impact on quit rates. Based on these findings, the researchers concluded that the nicotine patch is an effective aid for smoking cessation and has the potential to improve public health significantly. In addition to its use as a patch, nicotine is also available in the form of gum, an inhaler, nasal spray, and lozenges to help with smoking cessation.[16]

Non-nicotine agents. In the past few years, other pharmacological agents have also been used to facilitate smoking cessation, and their relative effectiveness compared to nicotine has been under study. Among the non-nicotine agents, bupropion was the first drug approved, with cessation rates ranging from 10.5–24.4 percent, depending on the dose. Bupropion has been used as an antidepressant, as well as treatment for adult attention deficit disorder and some psychiatric conditions. In clinical trials, the combined use of bupropion and a nicotine patch has also been effective for smoking cessation. Another drug approved for the treatment of smoking addiction is Varenicline (*Chantix*) and it too proved effective in abstinence from tobacco.

The studies on the use of pharmacological agents in smoking cessation underscore their importance in effectively helping smokers to quit. Only a small percentage of smokers (6.4 percent on average) are able to stop smoking on their own, unaided. The first, and the most critical, step is for the habitual smoker to want to quit. Once that is established, the smoker, and preferably his or her family or support system, should seek intervention from a healthcare provider and be actively involved in choosing which intervention to use. A close and consistent monitoring and follow-up by the healthcare provider is also critical for sustained success in overcoming this addiction to smoking. Even when the person's attempts fail to achieve the goal of abstinence, a retrial is advisable, as the prior attempts attest to the person's willingness and motivation to quit smoking. During the cessation attempts, the smoker should avoid such triggers to smoke as being in the company of smokers or drinking alcohol, as it lowers inhibition and prompts actions the smoker might otherwise abstain from. From a public health perspective, healthcare providers bear primary responsibility for identification and diagnosis of nicotine dependence, and initiating a discussion about smoking cessation and providing referral to an appropriate program.

There is generally a widespread recognition, even among smokers, that smoking is detrimental to health and wellbeing, and that the associated individual and societal costs are steep. Whether or not smokers perceive the specific risks of smoking and the benefits of quitting is another issue. A group of researchers sought to explore the association between smokers' perception of the risks of smoking and the benefits of quitting, and the extent to which these associations varied by demographic and other characteristics. The hypothesis in this relatively small study of 144 smokers was that a greater perceived risk of smoking would be associated with greater perceived benefits to quitting, and would be strongest among smokers who are concerned about the health effects of smoking and are motivated to quit. The findings revealed that smokers perceived themselves at risk for lung cancer regardless of whether they continued smoking or quit. This perception was strongest for older smokers who minimized the importance of reducing the lung-cancer risk, and was weakest for light smokers, African Americans, and smokers with higher intrinsic motivation for quitting relative to extrinsic motivation. The subgroup differences in perceptions of risks and benefits found in the study could be important to consider in education for smoking cessation.[17]

Many smokers contemplating quitting might want to know how soon after quitting can they expect to realize the benefits. Relative to current smokers, the documented health benefits gained by former smokers are significant and varied as follows: a 50-percent reduction in the risk for coronary heart disease at one year after quitting; a 60-percent reduction in risk for a major coronary event for men, and 70-percent reduction for women at three years; a reduction in risk of cancers of the mouth, throat, and esophagus by 50 percent at five years; and the risk for lung cancer, and death from chronic obstructive pulmonary disease (COPD) cut in half at ten years. Fifteen years after quitting smoking, the risk for coronary heart disease drops to nearly the same level as someone who never smoked. These are major health benefits gained at reasonably short intervals after stopping smoking, and should serve as powerful incentives for current smokers to quit smoking.[18]

Non-pharmacological Aids to Help Stop Smoking

E-Cigarettes. Electronic cigarettes (e-cigarettes) are battery-powered devices that deliver nicotine vapor without any combustion or smoke. Electronic cigarettes have gained popularity among smokers as a surrogate to cigarettes while attempting to quit smoking. However, due to concerns with poor manufacturing practices and the presence of known carcinogens in the limited products they tested, the United States Food and Drug Administration (FDA) has not approved or supported e-cigarettes for this purpose. A few studies have evaluated the effects of electronic cigarettes on nicotine levels and the heart rate, but have found negligible effects. Some surveys report success because users are able to cut back or stop the consumption of tobacco cigarettes, and only minor side effects, such as mouth and throat irritation, headache, vertigo, and nausea, have been noted. The scientific community, on the other hand, points out that the recruiting of participants in these surveys was done from e-cigarette Web sites, reflecting a bias, and that the tobacco cigarette use was self-reported by the participants rather than the nicotine levels being objectively tested. The studies that have formally evaluated nicotine craving when using electronic cigarettes yielded mixed results. More, and rigorous, studies on their safety and efficacy need to be completed in order to determine whether these products have a role in smoking cessation. E-cigarettes have been banned in some countries (e.g. Canada, Australia) due to a lack of definitive, credible evidence of their safety and efficacy.

Smokeless tobacco. The use of smokeless tobacco has reappeared in the United States, and is reported to be particularly popular among young white males, including school children. Oral snuff and chewing tobacco are the two most commonly consumed products.[19] The Food and Drug Administration (FDA) prohibits the sale of smokeless tobacco to individuals under the age of eighteen, and it imposes specific marketing, labeling, and advertising requirements. There is also evidence that the use of smokeless tobacco is a gateway to initiate smoking in young adult males. In one study, smokeless tobacco users were more than twice as likely to initiate, and smoke, cigarettes than nonusers, so smokeless tobacco use appears to be an important predictor of smoking initiation among young adult males. Based on their findings, researchers suggest that programs aimed at the prevention and cessation of smoking should also be extended to smokeless tobacco use.[20]

Drink Alcohol in Moderation or Not At All

There has been a great deal of research on the association between alcohol consumption and mortality from all causes, as well as from specific causes like heart disease and cancer. The association is often reported as a U- or J-shaped curve on a graph, meaning those who consume moderate amounts of alcohol have the lowest risk of mortality compared to both non-drinkers and heavy drinkers. Moderate consumption of alcohol has also been reported to have a protective effect against coronary heart disease. Questions have been raised about including non-drinkers in the research for comparison, as at least some of them may have stopped drinking because of an illness (resulting in estimates of artificially elevated rates of mortality among them), but most of the major studies controlled for this by including only disease-free (at the start) individuals in their study.

- A large study of Scottish men, with an unusually long follow-up of twenty-one years, was conducted in Scotland to determine the association between alcohol consumption and mortality from all causes, coronary heart disease, and strokes. The study started with 5,766 men employed at twenty-seven Scottish workplaces in Glasgow, Clydebank, and Grange Mouth between 1970 and 1973, when the men were between thirty-five and sixty-four years of age, and ended twenty-one years later. The participants reported if they drank alcohol, and if they did, the amount (spirits, beer, and wine) they consumed per week. For ease of comparison, the reported amount of alcohol consumed was converted into units, with 1 Unit equaling one shot of spirits, one pint of beer, or one-sixth a bottle of wine. The units of alcohol consumed per week were divided into six categories, from zero (non-drinkers) to thirty-five or more per week (heavy drinkers). The risk for all-cause mortality was similar for non-drinkers (zero units) and men drinking up to fourteen units a week. After that, the risk of mortality among drinkers rose with the increasing units of alcohol consumption, with men drinking thirty-five units or more per week doubling their risk of mortality. Overall, the risk of all-cause mortality was higher in men drinking twenty-two or more units (the equivalent of twenty-two shots of spirits) a week. There was a strong relation between alcohol consumption and the risk of mortality from stroke—men who drank thirty-five or more units had double the risk of non-drinkers, even after adjustment for other factors. In this study, there was no strong relationship shown between alcohol consumption and mortality from coronary heart disease.[21]

- In the past few decades, multiple studies in diverse populations have reported an inverse association between moderate alcohol intake and coronary heart disease. The studies pointed out that both men and women who consume one to three drinks a day have a 10–40-percent lower risk of coronary heart disease than those who abstain or drink more than three drinks a day. The risk is reported to increase incrementally in men and women who consume more than three drinks.

- The reduction in risk from moderate drinking is generally attributed to alcohol's beneficial effects for raising high-density lipoprotein (HDL). Researchers from the Harvard University School of Public Health and the University of California School of Medicine, San

Diego, performed a meta-analysis of forty-two pooled experimental studies that assessed the effects of moderate alcohol intake on concentrations of high-density lipoprotein cholesterol (HDL). Only men and women free of previous chronic disease were included in the studies, and the biomarkers were assessed before and after participants consumed up to, but not exceeding, 100 g of alcohol a day during the experimental study period. The findings revealed that a dose of 30 g of alcohol (the equivalent of one shot of spirits, one five-ounce glass of wine or two beers) increased concentrations of HDL to a level associated with an estimated 24.7 percent reduction in the risk of coronary heart disease. The researchers found other changes in biomarkers associated with an improved thrombolytic (blood-clotting factors) profile of the participants who drank alcohol, which they believe also contributed modestly in their risk reduction for coronary heart disease. Based on their findings, the researchers concluded that moderate alcohol consumption is causally related to lower risk of coronary heart disease.[22]

A word of caution is in order here for anyone currently abstaining from alcohol, but considering drinking it for its health benefits. Alcohol is a drug and can be habit-forming, and since some people are more prone to developing dependency than others, it is vital to carefully consider the risks and benefits of alcohol before starting to drink it for its health benefits alone. The benefits derived from moderate consumption of alcohol, such as a rise in HDL, can also be attained by regular exercise and other means. Furthermore, alcohol consumption beyond moderation (no more than one drink a day for women and two for men) is associated with a range of health problems, including obesity (central obesity in particular), heart disease, diabetes, and some cancers.

Based on what is known about the association between alcohol consumption and chronic disease risks, the key takeaway message is fourfold:

1. If you are currently an abstainer, you would be better off continuing to abstain and get the health benefits of moderate alcohol consumption in other ways, such as eating healthy, and exercising.

2. If you are a moderate consumer of alcohol, make sure you remain at that level of consumption and don't exceed it.

3. If you habitually drink more than what is regarded as moderate, scale back to the level of recommended moderation (no more than one drink a day for women and no more than two a day for men).

4. If you are a problem drinker (are alcohol dependent), seek professional help to overcome the problem and avoid a relapse.

Get Six to Seven Hours of Sleep in a Twenty-Four-Hour Period

With the increasing demands at work and home, the time adults spend asleep has steadily fallen in the United States. The average sleep duration among American adults in a recent poll was 6.9 hours per night, and 39 percent of the respondents slept less than 7 hours.[23] Many who sleep less than eight hours think they are not sleeping long enough, as they believe that eight hours of sleep in a day is essential for maintaining good health. There is, however, no scientific basis to justify recommending everyone get eight hours of sleep, or more, in a day. Sleep researchers and clinicians have been trying to determine if there is an optimal amount of sleep you should get in a day that would be beneficial for your health and be associated with the lowest mortality risk.

• As far back as 1959–1960, one million adult Americans who were participating in the Cancer Prevention Study I were surveyed about their sleeping patterns and were followed for six years into the future. Women and men who reported sleeping seven hours experienced the lowest mortality and a higher mortality was found among those who reported sleeping for eight hours or longer.

• These findings were also corroborated by the prospective study of Sleep Duration and Mortality Risk in Women among participants in the Nurses Health Study done from 1986–2000. During the fourteen years of this study, 5,409 deaths occurred in the 82,969 nurses who participated. The mortality risk was lowest among nurses reporting an average of seven hours of sleep per night. After adjusting for variables, the mortality risk for women sleeping five hours or less was found to be 15 percent greater than for those sleeping seven hours, while sleeping nine or more hours was associated with a 42-percent increase in mortality risk.[24] These results also confirm previous findings that the mortality risk in women is lowest among those sleeping six to seven hours. The finding in this study that the risk from increased sleep times (nine or more hours) was much greater than the risk attributable to reduced sleep times is also consistent with previous findings in other studies.[25]

- In a ten-year follow-up of a national cohort of 7,844 adults who participated in the First National Health and Nutrition Examination Survey (NHANES), researchers sought to find out if habitual sleep patterns were associated with increased risk for stroke and coronary heart disease. The results of their study showed that the risk for stroke was 1.5 times greater in those who reported sleeping longer than eight hours a night compared with those who slept between six to eight hours. In the same study, a similar relationship was also found between the duration of sleep and coronary heart disease, but it was weaker and did not reach statistical significance.[26]

Complaints of an inability to fall asleep (insomnia) are often indicative of other health problems, the most common one being depression. Indeed, when presented with sleep complaints, physicians diagnose depression more often than insomnia. Working on shifts is also reported to be a common cause of insomnia and reduced-sleep duration because of both circadian influences and environmental cues of attempting to sleep at irregular times. Regardless of the cause, any sleeplessness over a prolonged period requires medical attention, and intervention should be sought as promptly as possible. From the available evidence on the link between sleep duration and health, the clear message seems to be that the optimal amount of sleep everyone should try to get in a day is between six and seven hours. Less than five hours of sleep, or more than eight are both associated with negative health outcomes, including some serious ones, such as cardiovascular disease and stroke.

Manage Your Stress Effectively

Stress is defined in many different ways, but one definition offered by Professor Lazarus of the University of California, Berkeley in 1966, has endured, and is useful as it can be relevant in all contexts. According to Lazarus, "Stress occurs when an individual perceives that the demands of an external situation are beyond his or her perceived ability to cope with them."[27] Stress is experienced as a physiological, psychological, and emotional response to a stressor in the environment. Stressors can be factors or situations that are perceived to be good or bad. For example, fear of losing your job or receiving a job promotion can both generate stress. Ineffective coping can turn stress into distress that can have adverse effects on health, especially if continued over an extended period. Stress begins in the brain in response to a stressor, and affects the rest of the body. It can be acute, like that experienced in response to major events, such as the death of a loved one, being diagnosed with a catastrophic illness, divorce or break up from a long-term relationship, job loss, personal bankruptcy, or an environmental disaster (a house fire, flood, or earthquake). Stress can also be chronic from continued exposure to non-acute but lasting stressors, such as job stress, perception of unfair treatment by others, marital discord, financial problems, daily hassles like worsening rush hour traffic, and similar. Acute stress responses promote adaptation and survival via responses of the neural, cardiovascular, nervous (autonomic), immune, and metabolic systems. Chronic stress can promote or exacerbate abnormal changes through the same systems.

A physiological response to stress often kicks the body into a higher gear, and impulses signal the heart to beat harder and faster, cause blood pressure and pulse rate to rise, stimulate increased activity in the stomach and intestines (often described by people as a knot in the stomach), and trigger stress hormones to release more glucose, making more energy available to the brain and muscles. A psychological response often involves assessing the situation and its impact, and, depending on whether the stressor at hand represents a threat or a challenge, an emotional response can run the gamut of anger, sadness, resentment, disappointment, or joy. Stress is also very subjective, as an identical event can evoke an entirely different response from different individuals. Nevertheless, psychologists and psychiatrists have developed methods to evaluate and quantify stress levels based on generally agreed-upon rules for how stressful most people consider a given event.

The association between psychosocial stress and atherosclerotic events, such as coronary heart disease and myocardial infarction, has been the subject of many studies in the past twenty years. There has also been much written about the association between type-A behavior (driven, aggressive, impatient), high levels of job stress, and symptoms of coronary artery disease. One theory is that the correlation is determined by the response of the cardiovascular system to chronic stress (unabated stress over a prolonged period) that triggers *atherogenic* (plaque-generating) processes. In turn, these processes cause or exacerbate existing damage to the lining of the arterial wall, promoting atherosclerosis (hardening of the arteries). Research on stress and cardiovascular disease has shown that coping strategies play a major role in determining the impact of a stressor. Chronic stress is often associated with unhealthy behaviors, such as smoking, physical inactivity, and overeating.

- The INTERHEART study, a multinational study involving fifty-two countries and 25,000 people examined the relation of chronic stress to the incidence of myocardial infarctions (MI). All else being equal, the participants in the study who reported "permanent stress" at work or at home had greater than twice the risk of developing an MI compared to those who did not report such stress.[28] This finding is consistent with other epidemiologic studies that found individuals with high-stress jobs (high demands and low control) are at increased cardiovascular risk. Furthermore, studies have suggested that people who are chronically job-stressed may respond poorly to stressors outside the job.

- A relatively new environmental stressor facing millions of Americans is caregiving for an older family member. One of the most challenging scenarios for caregiving involves taking care of a parent or spouse with dementia, which can be physically and mentally draining for the caregiver. In one study, two researchers followed 400 caregivers and 400 matched non-caregiver controls over a four-year period to study the health effects of caregiving.[29] The caregivers had more sleep disruption, higher blood pressure, and higher inflammatory factors in their blood, and they experienced a 63-percent higher mortality than their non-caregiving counterparts.

Stress in itself is unavoidable as stressors can come from anywhere in the environment. The response to stress can, however, be modified so it doesn't adversely affect your health and wellbeing. There are approaches to stress management that can minimize the adverse effects of stress, and improve the morale and overall health and wellbeing of a person during times of stress. These include behavioral therapy, pharmacological aids, or a combination. Overall, the behavioral interventions are considered superior as they not only effectively improve coping with stress, but, unlike medications, they have no side effects. Behavioral therapies commonly used include biofeedback, cognitive behavioral therapy, meditation, and progressive relaxation. Prevailing science considers these interventions effective in coping with stress, improving overall wellbeing, and lowering blood pressure. A combination of two or more of these techniques has been found to have the most beneficial effect relative to any single intervention.[30]

- Cognitive behavioral therapy (CBT) has been extensively studied and found effective in the treatment of a variety of behavioral disorders, such as mood and anxiety disorders, obsessive-compulsive disorder, panic disorder, social phobia, post-traumatic stress disorder, depression, childhood depressive anxiety disorders, and anger management. It has also been tried successfully in the treatment of stress and stress-related illnesses. CBT is aimed at changing perceptions about stressors and reinforcing active coping skills. It may use different techniques, such as biofeedback, systematic desensitization, assertiveness training, and relaxation training, or a combination of them. CBT is generally short-term, averaging approximately eight to twelve sessions, meeting once or twice a week.

- Biofeedback is a technique designed to develop an individual's ability to control the autonomic nervous system that regulates heart rate, blood pressure, body temperature, and muscle tension. The person receives cues from a monitoring device when changes in these physiological parameters occur, and practices the behavioral technique to reverse the changes to the desired levels. In an experimental study to develop and test computer-aided biofeedback games to teach deep relaxation to patients with a stress-related illness, researchers in the U.K. found the technique effective in reducing the symptoms of illness.[31] The participants in this study were all diagnosed with irritable bowel syndrome, a condition known to be stress-related. Most participants learned to achieve progressively deeper levels of relaxation after four thirty-minute biofeedback sessions. At long-term follow up, nearly two thirds of the participants who had been helped by this relaxation technique continued to use the technique.

- Relaxation therapy has been successfully used either by itself or in conjunction with pharmacological agents in the treatment of illnesses in which stress is one of the associated factors, such as high blood pressure, and coronary heart disease.

- In experimental trials, meditation, yoga, and tai chi have been found to be very advantageous in the treatment of stress-related illnesses. In a Swedish study, a stress-management program based on cognitive behavioral therapy principles was compared with a *kundalini* yoga program.[32] The results showed that both cognitive behavior therapy and yoga are effective stress-management techniques. In the ancient practices of meditation, yoga, and tai chi, the central component of relaxation has long been associated with improved physiological and psychological wellness. For some time, there has been an increasing interest in these ancient techniques, meditation in particular, which has garnered evidence-based support for its therapeutic benefits. A meditation-inspired technique called mindfulness-based stress reduction (MBSR), originally developed by a professor at the University of Massachusetts Medical School, is based on mindfulness-meditation techniques that have been practiced in some form or another for centuries. This non-religious, and non-esoteric practice is aimed at enhancing awareness of the moment-to-moment experience of perceptible mental processes. It is believed that greater awareness will enhance perception, reduce negativity, and improve vitality and coping. In the last two decades, the use of this practice has been reported in many scientific journals, and has gained support for its use as a therapeutic aid in stress reduction and other related conditions to improve coping.[33] Research has shown that mindfulness practice has a demonstrable effect on the brain, the autonomic nervous system, stress hormones, and the immune system, and it can positively influence health behaviors, including eating, sleeping, and substance use.[34]

- It is also known that stress reduction often occurs when people indulge in activities they find pleasurable and satisfying. It's an undisputed fact that regular exercise of at least moderate intensity contributes to physical fitness, but there is also empirical evidence that exercise contributes to overall wellbeing, including psychological wellbeing. Studies have shown that exercise, both by itself and in combination with other interventions, can help alleviate the adverse effects of stress. The overarching implication is that a sense of wellbeing, both physiological and psychological, increases a person's ability to cope with stressors, and diminishes the adverse effects of stress on health.

- The pharmacological approach to stress management is generally based on countering the physiological and psychological responses to acute stress, by blunting or lessening the negative effects on the individual's coping ability. After fully assessing the individual's circumstances, the healthcare provider may select the appropriate drug or combination of drugs. Self-medicating is not advisable as it may not bring about the desired results, and could indeed cause harm.

Surround Yourself with a Strong Support System

There is much evidence that supportive social relationships have a major impact on both physical and mental health. Some even argue that social factors, such as socioeconomic status and social support, play even a larger role than factors like diet and exercise as "fundamental causes" of disease, because they embody access to important resources, affect disease outcomes in many ways, and are consequently linked to disease, even when intervening mechanisms change.[35] Research has linked the beneficial effects of social support to physiological processes within the cardiovascular, endocrine, and immune systems. There is also strong evidence that social integration leads to reduced mortality risks and a better state of mental health. Researchers believe the benefits of social support are primarily related to its stress-buffering effects, and its emotional support. It may also take other forms, like financial support or shared caregiving. Studies on social support point to the importance of familial support. But it is important to note here that the contemporary family is defined as whoever an individual considers his or her family to be, and is not necessarily confined to the traditional concept of a family related by blood or marriage—a modern family may not resemble a traditional family in its composition, but it does so in its function, especially with respect to serving as a support system.

- In a national study of marital status and mortality, researchers compared the death rates among married, widowed, divorced/separated, and never-married men and women, ages forty-five years and over.[36] Among the 281,000 participants in the study, each of the three non-married groups showed significantly higher death rates relative to the currently married group, ranging in relative risk from 1.24–1.39 in white men, 1.46–1.49 in white women, 1.27–1.57 in black men, and 1.10–1.36 in black women. The term *relative risk* is a ratio that compares the risk of disease (or death) in two groups, with 1.0 being the base point. The numbers here indicate that non-married white women and black men are at highest risk of death relative to their married counterparts. The mortality differential in the groups, referred to as the *marital advantage,* is attributed to the benefits of the built-in support system of married couples. With respect to the terms marriage and marital status, what should be underscored is the importance of their social support and their impact on health. Social support is also derived from other forms of committed relationships or strong personal friendships.

While social integration is generally associated with better health outcomes, the social relationships of a person represent a complex and dynamic network. Available data suggest that the quality of the social relationships influence the extent of these benefits—having 800 Facebook friends probably doesn't do the trick as they are not likely to be relationships that can be relied on for strong social support when needed. In contrast to the beneficial effects of social support, research has also shown that social isolation and non-supportive social interactions can have adverse effects on health, such as a lower immune function that can slow recovery from an illness.[37]

The next chapter will focus on the prudent use of preventive health services, including timely screening for early detection of disease that would help preserve and protect your health through risk assessment and timely intervention.

9

Regular and Effective Use of Preventive Health Services

In the previous chapter, lifestyle choices associated with good or bad outcomes in chronic diseases and overall health in general were described in some detail. The intent was to empower the readers with pertinent information, supported by scientific evidence, and promote lifestyle choices that lead to good health.

In this chapter, we will outline the currently available, evidence-based preventive health services that are aimed at protecting your health by assessing your risk for one or more chronic diseases, and providing you with appropriate intervention to prevent or delay their onset. And if a disease has already set in, preventive health services help detect it early in the disease process so that further progression is halted, and there is a better chance for reversal and recovery. In 1985, the Agency for Healthcare Research and Quality (AHRQ) convened the U.S. Preventive Services Task Force (USPSTF) to develop guidelines for evidence-based preventive services for groups at risk based on age, gender, and exposure to a range of diseases. The specific charge of the USPSTF was to rigorously evaluate available research-based evidence, and determine what clinical preventive services (e.g. screening tests, immunizations, prophylactic medications) are most effective and appropriate for different age and gender groups, taking into consideration their respective risks and benefits. The USPSTF is an independent panel of experts in primary care medicine and disease prevention, and uses most current scientific evidence to base their guidelines for effective preventive services across the lifespan, beginning with the pre-natal phase. Only those pertaining to adults and the chronic diseases described in this book are addressed here.

The USPSTF categorizes its recommendations based on a level of certainty (high, moderate or low) about the net benefit of a preventive measure to the individual at his or her risk level for a given disease. When the available evidence supporting the use of a preventive service gets consistently positive results from well designed and well-conducted scientific studies in representative populations, the task force deems the level of certainty about the net benefit of that service to be high. It regards the level of certainty moderate when the available evidence is derived from a limited number or size of studies, when the findings are inconsistent across studies, there are gaps in the chain of evidence, information is insufficient to assess effects on health outcomes, and findings are not generalizable to all populations. The USPSTF associates the net benefit of a preventive service with a low level of certainty when the available evidence is insufficient to assess the effects on health outcomes, or when the source of evidence on which it is based has important flaws in a study's design, methods, or other weaknesses. Based on the level of certainty about the net benefit of a preventive service, the USPSTF designates each of its recommendations as *A, B, C, D,* or *I*. The first two letters (*A* and *B*) signify that the task force found scientific evidence it regards as high or moderate enough to justify the recommendation. A recommendation is labeled *C* when the task force makes no recommendation for or against providing a particular preventive service because the balance of benefits and harms from the procedure is too close to justify recommending it. A designation of *D* to a recommendation means the task force is against routinely providing a particular preventive service to people without any manifestation (symptoms) of a disease because the evidence either points to the service being ineffective or being one where the harms outweigh the benefits. Lastly, a recommendation with an *I* designation simply means the task force concluded there is insufficient evidence to recommend for or against routinely providing a particular preventive service. These letter designations are particularly relevant in implementing the Affordable Care Act, for the law mandates that the recommendations the task force designated **A** or **B** are to be covered by the insurance at no charge to the patient.[1]

In addition to the recommendations by the task force, leading medical groups dedicated to the prevention and treatment of specific diseases, such as the American Heart Association (AHA), American College of Cardiology (ACC), American Cancer Society (ACS), American Diabetes Association (ADA), American College of Obstetrics and Gynecology (ACOG), and many others, offer their own guidelines, based on evolving scientific findings, and prevailing expert opinions in their respective fields. Occasionally, the two (USPSTF and a specialty medical group) sets of recommendations regarding a preventive service protocol for a particular chronic disease may be inconsistent with one another. Your primary physician would be able to sort out these differences, and select the best option based on your individual circumstances. Regardless of which recommendation is followed, they are all aimed at *risk assessment* and *risk intervention* for prevention or early detection of the diseases in question.

Despite these disease-prevention guidelines being available for several decades, the number of people benefiting from their utilization is woefully inadequate, reflecting a wide gap between the available knowledge and its practical utilization. Healthcare providers are urged to use every contact with their patients to explain, recommend, and follow up on the status of the recommended preventive action. Ultimately, however, the responsibility for carrying out the recommended action always rests with the individual, whether it's changing a health behavior or having a screening procedure done. Often, people do not give preventing the disease the same priority as having it treated once it sets in, even if preventing it means averting or stopping a potentially devastating disease in its tracks. This may be due to the fact that the effects of a disease that has not yet taken hold are not easy to fathom regardless of how devastating they could be, and especially if they are not receiving prompts and reminders from healthcare providers they trust and rely on for advice.

It is critical to follow your healthcare provider's age- and gender-based recommendations for disease prevention, and early detection, and if your provider does not initiate the conversation or make recommendations about screening tests appropriate for your age, gender, and risk profile aimed at early detection and intervention, it's in your best interest to bring the subject up and ask questions. For example, if you are a forty-year-old man or woman with a family history of colon cancer, you should have a conversation with your doctor about being screened for colon cancer, especially if the family member who had the disease was fifty-years-old or younger when diagnosed.

The recommendations are reviewed and revised on an ongoing basis as warranted by any new scientific findings. The guidelines are distributed to physicians across the country by the Agency for Healthcare Research and Quality (AHRQ), a division of the U.S. Department of Health and Human Services. Through multiple continuing medical education channels like professional conferences, lectures, and peer-reviewed professional journals, your healthcare provider is also kept abreast of the most recent, evidence-based guidelines and recommendations. With respect to the chronic diseases addressed in this book, a few examples of age- and gender-based preventive services currently recommended by the task force and/or a major specialty group are described below so you may understand why a particular recommendation may or may not apply to you in your particular set of circumstances. Be aware of the fact that even by the time this book goes into print, some of the recommended protocols currently in use may have been modified or replaced altogether in light of newfound scientific evidence. You can obtain information about the latest recommendation relevant to your risk profile from your physician or by going to the AHRQ website: www.ahrq.gov/clinic/uspstf/uspstopics.htm.

CARDIOVASCULAR DISEASE—SCREENING AND PREVENTION

1. The USPSTF and the American Academy of Family Physicians (AAFP) both recommend screening for *dyslipidemia* (abnormal cholesterol levels) only in those who are twenty years or older and at increased risk for heart disease. An assessment of your individual risk begins with obtaining your family history of the following diseases—coronary heart disease, high blood pressure or stroke, type-2 diabetes, and obesity. A positive family history of any of these places you at increased risk for one or more of them. You may also be tested for your baseline fasting blood-glucose level. These tests are repeated every five years for average-risk individuals, and every two years for those at high risk. A change, especially one that is significant in any of the measurements revealed by the test results, are discussed with you along with the implications of an elevated risk for the disease, and steps to reverse the change and stop it from recurring are recommended.

Your exposure to other major risk factors for cardiovascular disease, such as your smoking status, dietary habits, physical activity, and alcohol consumption, is assessed and documented, and in future visits, any subsequent changes in your exposure to these is noted. If you smoke, its adverse effects on your general health, and your cardiovascular health in particular, are explained to you; you are advised to quit and your willingness and readiness to quit is assessed. When you are ready, the available options for quitting are discussed. You are assisted with your choice, the appropriate referral to a smoking-cessation program is made with your cooperation, and your progress in stopping is monitored.

If your diet history indicates that you don't eat healthily, are overweight, and don't get enough exercise, you are informed of the negative consequences of these behaviors and are advised to modify them in favor of healthier ones. You are offered assistance and support in the process, including a referral to a dietitian or nutritionist if you wish. Your progress is assessed at each subsequent visit to your healthcare provider.

2. More recently, the American College of Cardiology and the American Heart Association have proposed a new tool for assessing an individual's ten-year risk of developing a fatal or nonfatal heart attack, a stroke, or another cardiovascular-disease event. While the tool and the concept it's based on are new, the risk factors it uses to determine the ten-year risk have long been recognized and include age, gender, race, cholesterol levels (all components), type-2 diabetes, smoking status, and blood pressure. This tool has thus far been tested only in select population groups—non-Hispanic whites and African-Americans. In predicting risk in the general population, however, the tool is reported to not be performing any better than other tools in validation studies. Taking this information into account, the American College of Cardiology and the American Heart Association guidelines suggest evaluating the risk factors for atherosclerotic cardiovascular disease every four to six years in individuals from twenty to seventy-nine years of age who do not have the disease, and using the new tool to calculate the ten-year risk for an event like a fatal or nonfatal heart attack or stroke in people from forty to seventy-nine years of age. Depending on your age, you may want to bring this up for discussion with your physician.[2]

3. The USPSTF recommends the use of low-dose (81 mg) aspirin for the Prevention of Cardiovascular Disease in men ages forty-five to seventy-nine years, and women ages fifty-five to seventy-nine, when the potential benefit of a reduced chance of a myocardial infarction outweighs the potential harm of an increase in gastrointestinal bleeding. This is a *Grade A recommendation* covered under the Affordable Care Act (ACA).

The task force recommends against the use of aspirin for stroke-prevention in women younger than age fifty-five, and for prevention of myocardial infarction (MI) in men younger than forty-five years of age. This is a *Grade D recommendation.*

The task force concludes that the current evidence is insufficient to assess the balance of benefits and harms in the use of aspirin for preventing cardiovascular disease in men and women ages eighty years or older, and thus does not recommend for or against it (*Grade I statement*).

The American Heart Association (AHA) acknowledges the proven value of low-dose aspirin in the treatment of an acute MI, as well as its long-term use in people with a prior cardiovascular disease, and believes that more widespread use of aspirin in these categories will contribute to reductions in cardiovascular-disease morbidity and mortality. It does, however, also believe that additional data are needed from randomized clinical trials to recommend aspirin use as a primary prevention in apparently healthy people. Until then, the AHA believes the use of aspirin in the primary prevention of MI should remain an individual healthcare provider's judgment, and that aspirin therapy should always be an adjunct, not an alternative to management of other risk factors. Although the recommendations of the USPSTF for aspirin use are more nuanced in terms of age and gender specifications than the AHA recommendation, there is no major inconsistency in their respective recommendations on this subject.

TYPE-2 DIABETES—SCREENING AND PREVENTION

1. The USPSTF recommends screening for type-2 diabetes in adults without symptoms of diabetes, but with persistent blood pressure (either treated or untreated) greater than 135/80 mm Hg, *Grade B recommendation* covered under the Affordable Care Act.

2. The USPSTF maintains that the current evidence is insufficient to recommend for or against routinely screening adults who are not experiencing any symptoms for type-2 diabetes or have blood pressure of 135/80 mm Hg or lower. *Grade I statement.*

Clinicians may also use indications other than those mentioned above for diabetes screening, such as a family history of type-2 diabetes. If one or more indicators are present in your case, you are assessed for your risk exposure by doing the following.

A. Recording your blood pressure, ordering a blood lipid test, and measuring your body mass index and waist circumference. If one or more of these parameters are higher than the lower target level for at-risk individuals, intervention with behavior modification only, such as diet and exercise, or in combination with a drug of choice, are offered and discussed with you.

B. Ordering one of the blood tests used to screen for diabetes— fasting plasma glucose (FPG), commonly referred to as fasting blood sugar, the two-hour oral glucose tolerance test (OGTT), or the hemoglobin A1c (HBA1c). The American Diabetes Association (ADA) recommends repeating the FPG test on a separate day to confirm the diagnosis, especially if the first test results are close to, but not within, normal range, and the clinician strongly suspects you have diabetes based on his or her clinical judgment. If the results are negative, the ADA recommends repeating the test every three years, or at shorter intervals for high-risk individuals.

3. Regardless of the outcome of screening tests, or even if the clinician believes testing is not warranted at a given time, you are advised and encouraged to eat a healthy diet, exercise regularly, maintain a healthy weight, and avoid smoking, or plan to quit if you do, in order to prevent or forestall the development of diabetes. Compliance with these recommendations should be monitored more closely if you are at a higher than average risk for the disease, such as having a family history of type-2 diabetes.

LUNG CANCER—SCREENING AND PREVENTION

1. In adults ages fifty-five to eighty years that have a thirty-pack-a-year smoking history and currently smoke or have quit within the past fifteen years, the USPSTF recommends annual screening for lung cancer with low-dose computed tomography (CT). It further recommends that screening be discontinued once a person has not smoked for fifteen years or develops a health problem that substantially limits life expectancy or the ability to have curative lung surgery. *Grade B recommendation* covered under the ACA.

2. Based on the results of the National Cancer Institute's National Lung Cancer Screening Trial, the American Cancer Society (ACS) also recommends lung-cancer screening in apparently healthy adults aged fifty-five to seventy-four years who have at least a thirty–pack-a-year smoking history and who currently smoke or have quit within the past fifteen years. In doing so, the ACS has acknowledged the National Lung Screening Trial findings, which established that annual screening with low-dose computed tomography (LDCT) reduces lung-cancer mortality in specific high-risk groups and saves many lives. The ACS does emphasize the importance of shared decision-making between clinician and patient, with the patient being fully informed prior to the screening of the potential benefits, limitations (screening will not detect all lung cancers), and harms associated with screening for lung cancer with low-dose computed tomography. Those choosing to undergo screening for early lung-cancer detection must also be informed that the LDCT scanning procedure is associated with a relatively high rate of false positives, stemming from identification of benign (non-cancerous), non-calcified nodules, and that detection of a cancer by LDCT does not guarantee a person can avoid death from lung cancer. The American Cancer Society emphasizes that counseling to stop smoking should remain a high priority in discussions with current smokers, informing them of their continuing risk of lung cancer, and making sure they know that screening should not be viewed as an alternative to smoking cessation.[3]

BREAST CANCER—SCREENING AND PREVENTION

Mammography is the standard radiological method of screening for breast cancer in women, and is recognized as playing a key role in early detection of the disease. Over the years, there have been several improvements in mammography techniques, including the introduction of full-field digital imaging, and more recently, the 3-dimensional *tomosynthesis* that yields images of multiple, thin cross-sections of the breast structure without overlapping, allowing better visualization of the breast tissue. The U.S. Food and Drug Administration (FDA) approved *tomosynthesis* for use in clinical settings in 2011. A recent, multi-center study has found the use of *tomosynthesis* particularly beneficial when combined with digital mammography in detecting invasive cancers through improved visualization, while reducing false-positive results associated with conventional mammography.[4] Although the combined use of digital mammography and *tomosynthesis* does double the dose of radiation, the total amount still remains well below the limits set by the Food and Drug Administration for its safe use.

Prevailing Recommendations on Mammography

1. The United States Preventive Services Task Force (USPSTF) has gone on record saying that mammography in women under fifty years of age results in minimal reduction in breast-cancer deaths, and higher rates of false-positives (results suggestive of cancer when there is none), and recommends screening by mammography beginning at fifty years of age with discontinuation at seventy-five years of age. The American Academy of Family Physicians (AAFP) has adopted the same position on breast-cancer screening for women as well.

The American College of Obstetricians and Gynecologists (ACOG) initially recommended mammograms every one to two years starting at age forty, and annually beginning at age fifty. However, ACOG revised its breast-cancer screening guidelines in 2011, recommending that mammography screening be offered annually to women beginning at age forty, citing the following reasons for the revision.

- While women in their forties have a lower overall incidence of breast cancer compared with older women, the window to detect tumors before they become symptomatic is shorter on average in these women.

- The five-year survival rate is very high (98 percent) for women whose breast-cancer tumors are discovered at their earliest stage, before they are palpable and when they are small and confined to the breast.

- Annual mammograms in women in their forties offer a better chance of detecting and treating the cancer before it has time to spread than if they waited two years between mammograms.[5]

2. The USPSTF regards the available evidence insufficient to recommend for or against clinical breast examination by a healthcare provider, or breast self-examination by women. The ACOG however recommends annual clinical breast exams (CBE) for women ages forty and older, and every one to three years for women ages twenty to thirty-nine. Additionally, it encourages "breast self-awareness" for women ages twenty and older, instead of the traditional breast self-exam (BSE). The breast self-awareness concept is based on women understanding the normal appearance and feel of their breasts (but without a specific interval or systematic examination technique), so they are alert to any changes in their breasts, no matter how small, and report them to their physician. The ACOG endorses educating women ages twenty and older regarding breast self-awareness.

3. In families with a much higher than expected incidence of both breast and ovarian cancer, an inherited gene mutation (*BRCA1* and *BRCA2*) is strongly suspected, and is associated with a significantly increased (up to 25 percent or greater) risk of breast cancer. Women with a strong family history (one or more first-degree relatives—mother or sister) of breast or ovarian cancer, and women who were treated for Hodgkin's disease or exposed to radiation to the chest between ages ten and thirty years are also considered to be at increased risk for breast cancer. The USPSTF recommends enhanced breast-cancer screening for women at high risk for breast cancer that includes mammograms before age forty, more frequent clinical breast exams, and annual MRIs (magnetic resonance imaging). It does not, however, recommend a breast MRI for women at low or average risk of developing breast cancer. The ACS guidelines also state that women at increased risk of breast cancer might benefit from additional screening strategies beyond those offered to women of average risk, such as earlier initiation of screening, shorter screening intervals, or combining mammography with other screening tests, such as a breast ultrasound or MRI. The ACS recommends against MRI screening for women at low risk (a lifetime risk of 15 percent or lower).[6]

COLORECTAL CANCER—SCREENING AND PREVENTION

Colorectal cancer (CRC) can largely be prevented by the detection and removal of adenomatous (non-cancerous) polyps, and survival is significantly better when the cancer is diagnosed while still localized. The colorectal-cancer screening tests are aimed at both detecting the cancer early, and detecting adenomatous polyps that can be removed to lower the risk for cancer development. The tests fall into two broad categories. The first includes stool tests (gFOBT, FIT, and sDNA) for occult blood that are primarily effective at identifying cancer, and the second encompasses partial or full structural exams (flexible sigmoidoscopy, colonoscopy), which are effective in detecting both cancer and premalignant polyps. The two types of tests differ in complexity and accuracy for the detection of cancer and advanced tumors. Although some precancerous polyps may be detected by stool tests, the potential for prevention is both limited and incidental. Among adults fifty years of age and older, only about 10 percent report the use of the FOBT (fecal occult blood test) stool test, and the use is lower among people who are ages fifty to sixty-four compared to those sixty-five years and older.

The stool tests are useful in screening for colorectal cancer in average-risk adults. Each test has strengths and limitations related to accuracy, cost, convenience, potential for prevention, and risk of missed detection. Any positive results should be followed-up by a colonoscopy for more complete diagnostic evaluation. The choice of a screening test should be a shared decision between the healthcare professional and their informed patient who has been given complete information about the risks and benefits of each test.

Recommended Screening Protocols

1. The USPSTF recommends men and women at average risk (based on the incidence in the general population) be screened with a full structural exam beginning at age fifty years and, depending on the type of test used (flexible sigmoidoscopy or colonoscopy), repeated every five to ten years. The recommendation for people at higher risk is to initiate screening at an earlier age. The high-risk group includes those with a family history of colorectal cancer or polyposis (presence of one or more polyps in the colon) that was diagnosed in a first-degree relative before sixty years of age, a personal history of ulcerative colitis, or high-risk genetic syndromes like the Lynch syndrome.

2. From 2006 to 2007, the American Cancer Society, the US Multi Society Task Force on Colorectal Cancer, and the American College of Radiology all came together to develop consensus guidelines for the detection of adenomatous polyps and colorectal cancer in average-risk adults who are not experiencing any symptoms.[7] Based on your risk status (average or high risk) your healthcare provider (HCP) would be advising you as to when your screening should begin. On the other hand, if you just had your fiftieth birthday and your HCP has not yet talked to you about your colorectal-cancer screening, it would be prudent for you to initiate a conversation about it, and follow through with scheduling the test when advised.

A large randomized control study in the U.K., tested the hypothesis that a single flexible sigmoidoscopy screening between fifty-five and sixty-four years of age can substantially reduce the incidence of, and deaths from, colorectal cancer. More than 170, 000 men and women from fourteen different facilities were randomly assigned to the control group (no screening, with flexible sigmoidoscopy) or the intervention group (screening, with flexible sigmoidoscopy), and were followed for an average length of eleven years. The incidence of colorectal cancer among the intervention group was reduced by 23 percent, and the death rate was reduced by 31 percent, relative to the control group. The study also revealed a 50-percent reduction in the incidence of distal colorectal cancer (rectum and sigmoid colon) in the intervention group during the follow-up period of eleven years. The researchers concluded that flexible sigmoidoscopy is a safe and practical test, and when performed once between ages fifty-five and sixty-four, confers a substantial and long-lasting benefit. The findings of this large and rigorous study underscore the importance of getting screened for colorectal cancer during the age interval (ages fifty-five to sixty-four years) when it is most likely to strike.[8]

Bowel cleansing is necessary to prepare the colon for this test, and it is typically performed without sedation. If there is a polyp or tumor present or suspected, the patient is referred for a colonoscopy so the colon can be examined further, and a polyp, if present, can be removed with a special instrument attached to the scope. Colonoscopy is usually performed under conscious sedation. Sigmoidoscopy, followed by colonoscopy can identify 70–80 percent of the individuals with advanced lesions, and is credited with a 60–80-percent reduction in deaths from cancer in the area of the colon reached and visualized by the examination.

Barriers to Screening for Colorectal Cancer

The rates of screening vary by race, income, and level of education. Screening rates are lower among those without health insurance coverage, and recent immigrants. The cost associated with the screening tests, especially those involving endoscopy, a lack of awareness of the need for, and importance of, screening, and a lack of access to healthcare seem to be the most common barriers to a higher use of colorectal screening. The invasiveness of the endoscopy procedures, and the fear and feelings of embarrassment also serve as deterrents to getting it done. Studies point to different preferences for testing methods between patient and provider, which may impact the screening rates. Physicians typically recommend colonoscopy, whereas patients often prefer the less invasive and more privately done FOBT stool test, although even that is not often carried out. Studies have also shown that an inadequate emphasis on the importance of colorectal screening for those in the risk category, and a failure by physicians to recommend a screening procedure reduces the likelihood of screening among both the insured and the uninsured individuals.[9]

Conversely, reducing or eliminating structural barriers to screening through meaningful one-on-one discussions between eligible patients and their healthcare providers about the benefits and limitations of various testing options, followed by concrete actions such as handing out FOBT cards, with instructions for their use at home, or providing a referral for such other procedures as colonoscopy or flexible sigmoidoscopy have been reported to increase the likelihood of colorectal screening. Mailed reminders to those who are due for screening have also proven effective.

The Affordable Care Act (ACA, 2010), the relatively new healthcare legislation is expected to have a positive effect on colorectal cancer screening. It includes approximately 160 provisions that are intended to improve healthcare for people with cancer, greater access to colorectal-cancer screening being one of them. The provision covering colorectal-cancer screening states that *"all new private health plans are required to cover colorectal cancer screening tests with a US Preventive Services Task Force (USPSTF) rating of A or B without any out-of-pocket costs to patients."* Effective 2011, preventive services for Medicare enrollees, such as colonoscopies, will have no out-of-pocket costs and are exempt from deductibles. The deductible will be waived for colorectal cancer screening tests even when polyps are detected and removed. Similarly, states are given an incentive by way of a 1-percent increase in the Federal Medical Assistance Percentages for preventive services if they offer Medicaid beneficiaries all preventive services recommended by the USPSTF, which include colorectal screening.

OBESITY—SCREENING AND PREVENTION

The most commonly used screening test for obesity in adults is a body mass index (BMI) assessment, which is easy to perform and is a highly reliable measure as it closely correlates with body fat in adults. The cutoff point for diagnosis of obesity is a BMI value equal to or greater than 30, and the risk for associated diseases like the cardiovascular diseases and type-2 diabetes increases with incremental rise in the BMI value.[10] In addition to the BMI, waist circumference, and the waist-to-hip ratio are also used to assess central obesity, even among non-obese persons. A waist circumference greater than 35 inches (88 cm) in women, and greater than 40 inches (102 cm) in men is associated with a higher risk for a cardiovascular disease.[11] Even mild to moderate overweight in young adults is predictive of subsequent obesity, and warrants close monitoring and counseling for adoption of healthier behaviors.[12] A BMI equal to or greater than 40 is considered extreme obesity, sometimes referred to as morbid obesity, and is on the rise in the U.S., having risen from 3.9 percent in 2000 to 6.6 percent in 2010. Extreme obesity is more common (about 50 percent higher) in women than in men.[13] Bariatric surgery (gastric by-pass) is often recommended for this level of obesity, especially if obesity-related comorbid (co-existing disease) conditions are present.

Accurate and appropriate assessment of overweight and obesity in children and adolescents is an increasingly critical aspect of modern medicine, given the rising prevalence of this health problem, and the promise that proper assessment and intervention can offer in preventing the progression of childhood obesity into adulthood.[14] The BMI has become the standard tool of assessment as a reliable indicator of overweight and obesity in adults. Children, however, are not classified according to absolute levels of BMI, but according to the age- and sex-adjusted BMI percentiles based on national data. A child with an age- and sex-adjusted BMI between the 5th and 85th percentiles is classified as having a healthy weight; a child with a BMI between the 85th and 95th percentiles is overweight; a child with a BMI in the 95th percentile or higher is considered obese. In addition to quantitatively determining the weight category, it is critical to evaluate the complex behavioral factors that influence obesity in children and adolescents. Clinicians have to be aware of, and sensitive to, the negative body image and self-esteem issues that overweight engenders among children, and need to be cognizant of the challenges in accurately assessing childhood overweight and obesity and recommending appropriate interventions.

The high prevalence of obesity-related chronic diseases underscores the need to prevent and reverse obesity rather than just treat its associated disease conditions. Once a determination is made that an individual is obese, the adverse effects on health are explained to that person, and counseling to advise and support a change in diet, exercise, or preferably both, is initiated. The focus of behavioral interventions should be on assisting the obese individual to acquire the needed skills and motivation to achieve a steady and sustained weight loss. The affected individual and the family (or his/her support system) should be fully involved in discussing and planning the interventions with the healthcare provider, and the other allied professionals involved.

Ensuring that individuals are informed about, and act on, appropriate and timely preventive health services are a critical component of chronic disease prevention and early detection strategy. It is a joint responsibility of the individual and the healthcare delivery system, with societal support in the form of healthcare coverage policies, such as the one provided for in the Affordable Care Act.

10

The Economic and Human Costs of the Major Chronic Diseases

The prevailing healthcare delivery system in the U.S. waits for the individual to become ill enough to experience symptoms of a disease and then seek medical care. With its focus on care of the sick, some have called it the revolving-door phenomenon because the sick enter the system, get treated for the episode, and then get sent home, only to return later with either another episode of the same illness or a new one, and this process keeps repeating itself over and over.

At the start of this book, where the stages in the progression of a disease were described, the symptomatic stage, known as the clinical stage, is the third one in line, preceded by two earlier phases of the disease. The first of these, the susceptibility stage, involves the interplay of risk factors that are laying the foundation for later development of disease. During this phase, in most cases, the disease could be prevented from developing by using risk assessment and intervention directed at eliminating or minimizing exposure to the known risk factors. In epidemiological terms, this is known as the *primary prevention*, and from both the individual and the public health perspectives, it results in the most good. If the disease escapes notice in this first stage, then the next best chance of catching the disease comes during the second stage, the pre-clinical stage, known as the *secondary prevention* phase, when interacting risk factors have begun to cause abnormal changes in the body, but the changes have not yet manifested themselves in the form of symptoms (e.g. pain or other discomfort). At this point, the disease can be detected by a trained healthcare professional who combines a clinical evaluation with one or more diagnostic tests. Detecting and treating the disease in this second stage, when interventions are most effective and the prognosis is better, can lead to significant reductions in disability and premature mortality, as well as in the high costs associated with management of chronic diseases. This stage is still regarded as having considerable value from both the public health and economic (cost-saving) perspectives. However, in the existing healthcare system, most often the initial point of contact between a patient and a healthcare provider does not take place in either of these stages as the seemingly well individual does not feel the need to visit a doctor, and the healthcare system has no system in place to prompt an asymptomatic individual to undergo screening for one or more diseases he or she may be at risk for. Currently, most people get screened for one or more diseases they may be at risk for if they are already seeing a doctor for another ongoing health problem.

There certainly is intent to bring about a change in the prevailing health care delivery system. This is evidenced at the national level by the release of the Federal Initiative, Healthy People 2020 (first released in 2000 as Healthy People 2000, and revised every 10 years since), and the appointment of the U.S. Preventive Services Task Force in 1985. The latter makes recommendations for screening disease-free individuals based on age, gender, and other potential risk factors, with the goals of achieving primary and secondary prevention. Although modest gains have been made in several areas of the 10-year Federal Initiative's goals, with only 3 percent of healthcare dollars invested in prevention, and 97 percent invested in treating the sick, disease prevention remains an elusive goal at the present. Lifestyle factors, such as an unhealthy diet, physical inactivity, and smoking were identified decades ago as major risk factors for cardiovascular diseases, certain cancers, and diabetes. A great deal of research has been done, and many volumes have been written about effectively preventing and/or minimizing a person's exposure through lifestyle modification. Increasingly sophisticated screening and diagnostic procedures are available, along with evidence-based recommendations for their use according to age, gender, and other risk-based indications. Together, these measures can help achieve primary and secondary prevention of the burdensome chronic diseases to a far greater extent than is being done at present. The number of Americans living with preventable chronic conditions has reached an unprecedented level, along with an equally unprecedented level of associated healthcare costs for their treatment. Advances in technology, as well as more and better drugs, are also boosting the prevalence (the number of people living with a disease) rates of chronic diseases by making it possible for people with a chronic disease to live longer, although not necessarily disease-free. This is reflected in ever-increasing healthcare expenditures at all levels of society—federal, state, local, and individual.

Collectively, cardiovascular diseases (including stroke), cancer, and diabetes account for two-thirds of all deaths in the United States, and a third of the 2.8 trillion (in 2014 dollars) annual healthcare costs. The costs include both direct medical-care costs and indirect economic costs from lost productivity due to illness or death. The direct medical-care costs associated with a disease include the cost of physicians and other healthcare professionals, hospital and nursing home services, the cost of medications, and home healthcare. They do not include the costs of treating and/or managing health problems, impairments, functional limitations, or additional disabilities that are secondary to a chronic disease. For example, type-2 diabetes, if not well controlled, may give rise to heart disease, neuropathy, end-stage renal disease, blindness, and toe and lower limb amputations that generate additional treatment costs as well as personal hardship. In 2012, one in five healthcare dollars was spent on the care of people with diabetes, including treatment of the complications arising from the disease, at a total annual estimated cost of $245 billion (in 2012 dollars).[1] Similarly, while the annual direct costs associated with obesity as a chronic disease were estimated at $150 billion (in 2008 dollars), the costs of treating the conditions that are secondary to obesity, such as heart disease, diabetes, and certain cancers, far exceed that. The costs cited with respect to both chronic diseases mentioned above only refer to the direct costs, and do not include indirect costs caused by the person's lost productivity or those of the care-giving family members, which are estimated to be nearly four times that of the direct costs.

In a presentation made for a stakeholder forum in 2007, Ross Devol, Director of the Center for Health Economics at the Milken Institute, discussed the expected steep rises in the number of people living with a chronic disease in the twenty-year period from 2003 to 2023.[2] His projected rates of increase are staggering—62 percent for all cancers combined, 53 percent for type-2 diabetes, 41 percent for heart disease, and 29 percent for strokes. During the same period, the projected population growth was only 19 percent.[3] Devol also projects that the combined value of medical expenditures and productivity losses associated with chronic diseases in the U.S. will approach 4 trillion dollars by 2023, if the projected rates of increase in chronic diseases continue unabated, and the rising costs of healthcare are not reigned in.

People with chronic diseases account for a disproportionately large share of healthcare use, representing 69 percent of hospital admissions, and 80 percent of hospital days. Their average length of hospital stay is also longer than for those without chronic conditions (7.8 days vs. 4.3 days). As well, anyone with one or more chronic diseases incurs a disproportionately high number of home care visits, prescription drug use, visits to a physician, and emergency-department use. Medicare spending is heavily skewed toward enrollees with chronic diseases, the per-capita medical spending being three to ten times higher for older adults with one or more chronic conditions than for those without.[4]

The Magnitude of Chronic Diseases problem in the U.S.

Trends in incidence, prevalence, and mortality for chronic diseases are influenced by demographic shifts in the U.S. population, such as the aging of baby boomers (age is a non-modifiable risk factor). Among the fifteen leading causes of death in the U.S., published by the National Center for Health Statistics of the U.S. Department of Health and Human Services in 2013, heart disease and cancer continue to rank as numbers one and two respectively, stroke takes up the fourth place and type-2 diabetes the seventh. Despite a declining trend in the death rate from cardiovascular diseases, the number of deaths from cardiovascular causes continues to rise each year, accounting for one out of every three deaths.[5] This increase in the number of deaths is primarily attributed to an increase in the size of the population over the age of sixty-five years. Every year, over 735,000 Americans experience a first heart attack, and half as many experience a recurrent attack in the United States. Coronary heart disease (CHD) is the most common type of heart disease, killing over 370,000 people annually. Each year more than 795,000 people in the United States have a stroke, and 130,000 die from one each year accounting for 1 out of every 20 deaths, despite a significant decline (19.4 percent) in deaths from stroke in the two decades from 1988 to 2008.[6]

One in four adults in the U.S. has high blood pressure, and for a majority of them, the blood pressure is not adequately controlled, even with treatment.[7] Estimates from the Third National Health and Nutrition Examination Survey indicate that among individuals with health insurance, 28.6 percent of the adults with high blood pressure and 51.2 percent of the adults with abnormally high cholesterol level were undiagnosed.[8]

Few people with a chronic disease have it as their only disease condition; most also have one or more other chronic diseases. According to a brief released by the National Center for Health Statistics in 2010, 45% of adults had at least one of three diagnosed or undiagnosed chronic conditions—hypertension (uncontrolled high blood pressure), high cholesterol, or type-2 diabetes.[9] And one in eight adults (13%) had two of these conditions; and 3% of adults had all three chronic conditions. This is referred to as *multi-morbidity* (co-existence of multiple disease conditions) and is more commonly experienced among the older individuals, ages sixty-five years or older, although one in four adults who experience multi-morbidity is younger than sixty-five years of age. It has been reported that only 17 percent of those diagnosed with, for example, coronary heart disease, have it as the sole chronic condition with no other coexisting chronic disease.[10]

As can be expected, adults with multiple disease conditions use healthcare services more frequently than those without coexisting chronic conditions, and they account for two-thirds of the healthcare costs. Treating people with multiple disease conditions also poses added challenges to healthcare providers because they have to weigh treatment options so that any given treatment, while being beneficial in one condition, does not adversely affect another condition.[11] Having multiple co-existing diseases also adds to the burden of the patient, as he or she has to make frequent visits to the healthcare provider, likely take multiple drugs at different intervals, and endure other lifestyle limitations.

In the past twenty-five years, there has been a modest decline in the death rate from all cancers combined in the U.S. primarily due to a reduction in smoking rates and improvements in the early detection and treatment of cancers. However, as with cardiovascular diseases, the annual deaths from cancer increased due to both an increase in the total population, and a disproportionate increase in the group aged sixty-five years and older.Changes in lifestyle, screening for early detection, and improvements in treatment also affect trends and patterns in the prevalence of chronic diseases. The current rising trend in overweight and obesity rates, including among children, will likely add to the incidence and prevalence of chronic diseases in the future, and exacerbate the associated human and economic costs. Adding about 1.3 million new cases each year, the case in point is type-2 diabetes, which has increased by more than 60 percent in the past twenty-five years, corresponding to a rise in the prevalence of overweight and obesity.

Nearly one in five deaths from a chronic disease is among people aged forty-five to sixty-four years, well below the average life expectancy, and below the normal retirement age. This accounts for the loss of a substantial number of years of life, and the consequent productivity losses translate into a multi-billion dollar economic loss to society. In fact, as a source of economic burden, the costs of lost productivity from premature deaths attributed to chronic diseases are reported to have surpassed the costs of the diagnosis and treatment of these diseases. This is especially egregious since the illness, disability, and premature deaths are stemming from *preventable* chronic diseases. It is estimated that, by 2030, one in five Americans will be age sixty-five or older, and the number of those with chronic conditions will likely increase to 148 million, and will include a concomitant rise in the total direct and indirect costs associated with them.[12]

For the affected individuals and their families, the burden of living with a chronic disease can also be formidable due to the possible loss of income from increased time off from work for self and caregiver, possible increases in health insurance premiums, and increased out-of-pocket medical costs. The cost of such intangibles as pain and suffering, the inability to function within the family and society as a parent, husband/wife, breadwinner, and productive member of society, plus the reduced overall quality of life for self and family can be incalculable. Studies have shown higher rates of depression among those diagnosed with a chronic disease, especially one, such as a stroke, that can result in some loss of function temporarily or permanently. Other studies have documented significant levels of cognitive impairment following heart failure or cardiac surgery. Depression or poor cognitive functioning may, in turn, interfere with treatment compliance, and affect disease outcome. The disease takes a toll on many fronts, and for the affected individuals and their families, the human costs of living with a chronic disease are even greater than the economic costs.

The majority of those with chronic conditions are not disabled and do live normal lives, but they live with the threat of recurrent crises, higher healthcare costs, more days lost from work, and the risk of long-term limitations and disabilities. The high healthcare rates among those with one or more chronic diseases make them less attractive to insurers, and if they were not already insured prior to developing the condition, many insurers would not insure them, citing a pre-existing condition as the reason. This is no longer the case, but prior to the passing of The Affordable Care Act, this made switching jobs untenable for many who feared they would be uninsurable if they lost their current insurance. The high cost of insurance premiums also causes many to be underinsured, and carry high deductibles and out-of-pocket expenses that result in an increasingly larger portion of their income going toward medical expenses. It is not uncommon for a family with a high deductible to have to pay $20,000 or more in a year if they incurred large bills from costly procedures or one or more hospitalizations. These payments could, fairly quickly, put a middle-income ($40,000/year) family on the path to financial ruin, including, for some, being forced into bankruptcy. In terms of both economic and human costs, the burden of chronic diseases is high and rising. The major chronic diseases—heart disease, cancer, diabetes, and stroke—are robbing those affected of both years of life and years of *healthy* life.

Summary

The average lifespan in the industrialized countries has risen by nearly thirty years in the past 100 years. During that time, eradicating or greatly reducing the incidence of killer communicable diseases achieved the bulk of the gain in longevity. These gains have since been furthered by innovations in medical sciences, and advances in technology that have helped accelerate those innovations. However, non-infectious, killer chronic diseases that have reached epidemic proportions in the past decades are plaguing the years of life thus gained, and are increasingly responsible for poor health and premature deaths in the middle and later years. There is mounting scientific evidence associating such behaviors as smoking, not eating a healthy diet, being physically inactive, and being overweight with a substantial increase in a person's lifetime risk of developing, or dying from, a cardiovascular disease, type-2 diabetes, or some types of cancer. Yet, too many people still smoke, eat an unhealthy diet, and do not exercise regularly.

Chronic diseases have a long latency period as the foundation for their origin is often laid in early life by multiple, synergistic (interacting) risk factors, and the diseases themselves progress insidiously over many years or even decades. The rising incidence and prevalence of chronic diseases have spurred research related to their causes and prevention that has led to an unprecedented, and continually expanding knowledge base in this area. Researchers have been able to establish evidence-based links between an increased risk for development of a particular chronic disease and exposure to certain environmental, life-style, and genetic factors, often in quantifiable terms. This knowledge has aided in reducing the incidence of some of the chronic diseases like heart disease through mass educational campaigns to lower exposure to major risk factors. Reduction in smoking rates is a prime example of such an effort. Innovations in screening techniques, coupled with their use at optimal intervals based on risk profiles of individuals are also aiding in early detection and intervention that significantly improves the outcome in chronic diseases.

There are many risk factors within the control of the person that deter-mine whether he or she succumbs to a certain disease, able to keep it at bay for a lifetime or delay it for an extended period of time. These are referred to as the 'modifiable' risk factors because these can frequently be altered through *lifestyle* choices to mitigate their disease-causing capacity, whereas inherited risk factors are rarely modifiable and are thus termed 'non-modifiable' risk factors. Those that are modifiable through *lifestyle* choices include diet, physical activity, tobacco use, alcohol con-sumption, adequate rest and sleep, effective stress management, family and personal relationships, and finally, a prudent use of preventive health services. The amount, and the length (in years) of smoking, for example, not only increase the risk for diseases like lung cancer and emphysema, but also increase the person's susceptibility to other illnesses. Both a high fat diet and physical inactivity contribute to weight gain, which over time can put a person at an increased risk for diseases associated with overweight and obesity such as heart disease, adult-onset diabetes, high blood pressure, and some types of cancers.

The unprecedented gains in lifespan in the last century has also sparked questions and concerns about quality of life, especially in mid-dle and later years when chronic diseases are most likely to strike. Whether longevity and quality of life are mutually exclusive concepts or can and should co-exist are questions being increasingly raised in many parts of the world today. Many believe extension of healthy longevity marked by good health and vigor shortens the period of senescence that is characterized by reduced vigor and increased disability, near the end of life. Terms like "healthy life expectancy" and "healthy longevity," meant to convey a combination of the length and quality of life, are increasingly being used as a measure of population health.[1] Working toward an improvement in quality of life to keep pace with the increase in life expectancy is a health policy concern in many countries. The steadily rising health care costs, far exceeding the rate of inflation, and a lack of access to health care by a significant number of uninsured Americans has been the impetus for the health care reform efforts in the U.S. that led to the introduction of the Affordable Care Act in 2010. Extending the focus to outcome measures that takes into account both longevity and quality of life could help guide allocation of resources to the broader social and environmental determinants of health. This may be particularly critical in the face of burgeoning incidence and prevalence of chronic diseases like type-2 diabetes, obesity, cardiovascular diseases, and cancer in the U.S.

Chronic disease prevention requires investment on many fronts—the individual, the society, and the health care industry. At the individual level, it requires a reframing of thinking about lifestyle choices and chronic disease connection, as the disease may not surface for years or decades after exposure to risks. Available evidence unequivocally points to the fact that chronic diseases strike people with a particular set of lifestyle choices more often than those who do not make those choices, and as well that adopting healthier choices at any age, and stage of disease progression has proportional benefits. The society, for its part, needs to invest more resources like money and personnel, and put in place meaningful health policies, and secure a buy-in of those policies by the public and the healthcare providers, to improve public health through disease prevention, and health promotion. There is undoubtedly, a need for a cultural shift in the U.S. healthcare-delivery system to put disease prevention on the same footing as disease intervention so the demand for the latter is reduced over time, and more resources can be diverted to keeping people healthy instead of perpetuating a revolving door of sick care. Such a shift also calls for members of the health care delivery system to embrace disease prevention with the same zeal and passion as they do disease intervention. A commitment on the part of health care providers to seize every opportunity to educate the patient and his or her family about disease prevention, through healthy lifestyle choices, and the use of preventive health services goes a logway in preventing and/or postponing illness and death, as well as extending healthy longevity. This is especially relevant in chronic disease prevention, as these diseases have a long latency period and provide ample opportunities to facilitate adoption and/or modification of lifestyle choices that hold the most promise for prevention and/or early detection and intervention of the killer chronic diseases addressed in the book.

Endnote References

Introduction

1. Woolf, SH, Aron, LY. "The U.S. Health Disadvantage Relative to Other High-Income Countries: Findings from a National Research Council/Institute of Medicine Report." *The Journal of the American Medical Association (JAMA)*. 309(8):2013, 771-772.

2. Webber, BJ, Seguin, PG, Burnett, DG, et al. "Prevalence of and Risk Factors for Autopsy-Determined Atherosclerosis Among US Service Members, 2001-2011." *The Journal of the American Medical Association (JAMA)*. 308(12):2012, 2577–2583.

3. Murphy, SL, Xu, J, Kochanek, KD. "Deaths: Final Data for 2010, Centers for Disease Control and Prevention." *National Center for Health Statistics Reports*. May 8, 2013.

4. Buettner, Dan. *The Blue Zones, 2nd ed.: 9 Lessons for Living Longer from the People Who've Lived the Longest*. Washington, D.C: The National Geographic. 2012.

5. Breslow, L, Enstrom, JE. "Persistence of health habits and their relationship to mortality." *Preventive Medicine*. 9(4):1980, 469-483.

Chapter 1

1. Duncan, FD. *Epidemiology: Basis for Disease Prevention and Health Promotion*. New York, NY: Macmillan Publishing Company, 1988.

2. Huxley, R, Barzi, F, Woodward, M. "Excess risk of fatal coronary heart disease associated with diabetes in men and women: meta-analysis of 37 prospective cohort studies." *British Medical Journal*. 332(73):2006, 1–6.

Chapter 2

1. Mausner, JS, Kramer, S. *Epidemiology—An Introductory Text*. Philadelphia, PA: W.B Saunders Company, 1985.

Chapter 3

1. Paffenbarger, RS, Hyde, RT, Alvin, MA, et al."The Association of Changes in Physical-Activity Level, and other Lifestyle Characteristics with Mortality among Men."
New England Journal of Medicine. 328(8):1993, 538–545.

Chapter 4

1. Mozaffarian D, Benjamin EJ, Go AS, et al. "Heart disease and stroke statistics—2015 update: a report from the American Heart Association." *Circulation.*
131:2015, 322-329.

2. Kochanek, KD, Xu, JQ, Murphy, SL, et al. "Deaths: final data for 2009." *National
Vital Statistics Reports.* 59:2011, 1–8.

3. Lloyd-Jones, DM, Hong, Y, Labarthe, D, et al. "Defining and Setting National
Goals for Cardiovascular Health Promotion and Disease Reduction: The American
Heart Association's Strategic Impact Goal Through 2020 and Beyond." *Circulation.*
121:2010, 586–613.

4. Kromhout, D, Alessandro, M, Kesteloot, H, et al. "Prevention of Coronary Heart
Disease by Diet and Lifestyle: Evidence from prospective cross-cultural, cohort, and
intervention studies." *Circulation.* 105:2002, 893–898.

5. Timmreck, TC. *An Introduction to Epidemiology.* Boston, MA: Jones and Bartlett
Publishers, 1994.

6. Keys, A. *Seven Countries. A multivariate analysis of death and coronary heart
disease.* Cambridge, MA: Harvard University Press, 1980.

7. Ludwig, DS. "Examining the Health Effects of Fructose." *The Journal of The
American Medical Association (JAMA).* 310:2013, 33–34.

8. Boren, J, Gustafsson, M, Skalén, K, et al. "Role of extracellular retention of low density lipoproteins in atherosclerosis." *Current Opinion in Lipidology.* 11:2000, 451–456.

9. Li, S, Chen, W, Srinivasan, SR, et al. "Childhood Cardiovascular Risk Factors and
Carotid Vascular Changes in Adulthood: The Bogalusa Heart Study." *The Journal of
The American Medical Association (JAMA).* 290(17):2003, 2271–2276.

10. Go, AS, Mozaffarian, D, Roger, VL, et al. "Executive Summary: Heart disease
and stroke statistics—2013 update: a report from the American Heart Association."
Circulation. 127:2013, 143–152.

11. Simon, BH. "Meat or beans: What will you have? Part 1: Meat." *Harvard Men's
Health Watch.* 15:2011, 1–3.

12. Simon, BH. "Meat or beans: What will you have? Part I1: Beans." *Harvard Men's
Health Watch.* 15:2011, 4–6.

13. Samara, JN, Popkin, BM. "Patterns and Trends in Food Portion Sizes, 1977–1998."
The Journal of The American Medical Association (JAMA). 289(4):2003, 450–453.

14. US Department of Health and Human Services. *The biology and behavioral basis*

for smoking-attributable disease: A report of the Surgeon General. CDC, Atlanta, GA, 2010.

15. Doll, R, Peto, R. "Mortality in relation to smoking: 20 years' observations on male British doctors." *BMJ* (Formerly *British Medical Journal*). 2:1976, 1525–1536.

16. Centers for Disease Control and Prevention. Smoking-attributable mortality, years of potential life lost, and productivity losses, United States, 2000–2004. *MMWR (Morbidity and Mortality Weekly Report)*. 57(45):2008, 1226–1228.

17. Xu, X, Bishop, EE, Kennedy, SM, et al. Annual Health Care Spending Attributable to Cigarette Smoking: An Update. American Journal of Preventive Medicine. (Italicize) 48 (3):2014,326-333.

18. Kuulasmaa, K, Tunstall-Pedoe, H, Dobson, A, et al. "Estimation of the contribution of changes in classic risk factors to trends in coronary event rates across the WHO-MONICA Project populations." *The Lancet.* 355 (9205):2000, 675–687.

19. Ksaniemi, YA, Danforth, E, Jensen, MD, et al. "Dose-response issues concerning physical activity and health: an evidence-based symposium." *Medicine & Science in Sports & Exercise.* 33:2001, S351-S358.

20. Mitka, M. "Study: Exercise May Match Medication in Reducing Mortality Associated with Cardiovascular Disease, Diabetes." *The Journal of The American Medical Association (JAMA).* 310(19):2013, 2026–2027.

21. Thompson, PD, Franklin, BA, Balady, GJ, et al. "AHA Scientific Statement: Exercise and Acute Cardiovascular Events." *Circulation.* 115:2007, 2358–2368.

22. Centers for Disease Control and Prevention."Million Hearts: Strategies to reduce the prevalence of leading cardiovascular disease risk factors-United states, 2011." *MMWR (Morbidity and Mortality Weekly Report).* 60(36):2011, 248–1251.

23. Boden, WE, Franklin, BA, Wenger, NK. "Physical Activity and Structured Exercise for Patients with Stable Ischemic Heart Disease." *The Journal of The American Medical Association (JAMA).* 309(2):2013, 143–144.

Chapter 5

1. Reaven, GM. "Banting Lecture 1988: Role of insulin resistance in human disease." *Diabetes.* 37:1988, 1595–1607.

2. Anderson, PJ, Critchley, JH, Chan, CN, et al. "Factor analysis of metabolic syndrome: Obesity vs. insulin resistance as central abnormality." *International Journal of Obesity.* 25(12):2001, 1782–1788.

3. Weihang, B, Srinivasan, SR, Wendy, A, et al. "Persistence of Multiple Cardiovascular Risk Clustering Related to Syndrome X From Childhood to Young Adulthood: The Bogalusa Heart Study." *Archives of Internal Medicine.* 154(16):1994, 1842–1847.

4. National Institutes of Health. "How is metabolic syndrome diagnosed?" www. Mayoclinic.org. Retrieved 6/12/2014.

5. Ford, ES, Giles, WH, Dietz, WH. "Prevalence of the metabolic syndrome among

US adults: findings from the third National Health and Nutrition Examination Survey. *The Journal of the American Medical Association. (JAMA).* 287:2002, 356–359.

6. Beckman, JA, Creager, MA, Libby, P. "Diabetes and atherosclerosis: epidemiology, pathophysiology, and management." *The Journal of the American Medical Association (JAMA).* 287:2002, 2570–2581.

7. Lofgren, IE, Herron, KL, West, KL, et al. "Weight Loss Favorably Modifies Anthropometrics and Reverses the Metabolic Syndrome in Premenopausal Women." *Journal of the American College of Nutrition.* 24(6):2005, 486–493.

8. Galassi, A, Reynolds, K, He, J. "Metabolic Syndrome and risk of cardiovascular disease: a meta-analysis." *American Journal of Medicine.* 119:2006, 812–819.

9. Centers for Disease Control and Prevention. *National Diabetes Fact Sheet: National estimates and general information on diabetes and pre-diabetes in the United States, 2011.* Atlanta, GA: Centers for Disease Control and Prevention, 2011.

10. Geiss, LS, James, C, Gregg, EW, et al. "Diabetes Risk Reduction Behaviors among U.S. Adults with Pre-Diabetes." *American Journal of Preventive Medicine.* 38(4):2010, 403–409.

11. Ratner, R, Goldberg, R, Haffner, S, et al. "Impact of Intensive lifestyle and metformin therapy on cardiovascular risk factors in the diabetes prevention program." *Diabetes Care.* 28:2005, 888–894.

12. American Diabetes Association. "Diagnosis and Classification of Diabetes Mellitus." *Diabetes Care.* 33:2010, S62–S69

13. Bell, C, Kermah, D, Davidson, MB. "Utility of A1C for diabetes screening in the 1999–2004 NHANES population." *Diabetes Care.* 30(9):2007, 2233–2235.

14. Tuomilehtz, J, Lindström, J, Johan, G, et al. "Prevention of Type 2 Diabetes Mellitus by Changes in Lifestyle among Subjects with Impaired Glucose Tolerance." *The New England Journal of Medicine.* 344(5):2001, 1343–1350.

15. O'Keefe, JH, Bell, HD, Wayne, LK, et al. *Diabetes Essentials.* 2nd Ed. Royal Oak, MI: Physicians Press, 2005.

16. Edward, WG, Xiaohul, Z, Yilling, JC et al. "Trends in lifetime risk and years of life lost due to diabetes in the USA, 1985-2011: a modeling study." *The Lancet.* 2(11) 2014, 867–874.

17. Shaw, JE, Sicree, RA, Zimmet, PZ. "Global estimates of the prevalence of diabetes for 2010 and 2030." *Diabetes Research and Clinical Practice.* 87(1):2010, 4–14.

18. Goldstein, BJ, Miller, JL, Ahmad, I. *Contemporary Diagnosis and Management of The Patient With Type-2 Diabetes.* Longboat Key, FL: Handbooks in Healthcare, 2008, 54–55.

19. Kahn, SE. "The relative contributions of insulin resistance and beta-cell dysfunction to the pathophysiology of Type 2 diabetes." *Diabetologia.* 46:2003, 3–19.

20. American Diabetes Association. "Standards of Medical Care in Diabetes." *Diabetes Care.* 33(S1):2010, S11–S61.

21. Garber, AJ. "Treatment of Hypertension in Patients with Diabetes Mellitus." In Taylor SI, ed. *Current Review of Diabetes.* Philadelphia, PA: Current Medicine Inc., 1999.

22. Klein, R, Aiello, LP, Chiang, Y, et al. "The Wisconsin Epidemiologic Study of Diabetic Retinopathy. II. Prevalence and risk of diabetic retinopathy when age at diagnosis is less than 30 years." *Archives of Ophthalmology.* 102:1984, 520–526.

23. Meijer, JW, Trip, J, Jaegers, SM, et al. "Quality of life in patients with diabetic foot ulcers." *Disability and Rehabilitation.* 23:2001, 336–340.

24. Zimny, S, Schatz, H, Pfohl, M. "The role of limited joint mobility in diabetic patients with an at-risk foot." *Diabetes Care.* 27:2004, 942–946.

25. Pecoraro, RE, Reiber, GE, Burgess, EM. "Pathways to diabetic limb amputation: basis for prevention." *Diabetes Care.* 13:1990, 513–521.

26. Gregg, EW, Sorlie, P, Paulose-Ram, R, et al. "Prevalence of lower-extremity disease in the US adult population 40 years of age or older with and without diabetes: 1999-2000 National Health and Nutrition Examination Survey." *Diabetes Care.* 27:2004, 1591–1597.

Chapter 6

1. American Cancer Society. *Cancer Facts & Figures 2013.* Atlanta, GA: American Cancer Society, 2013.

2. Wiseman, M. "Food, Nutrition, Physical Activity, and the Prevention of Cancer: A Global Perspective." *Proceedings of the Nutrition Society.* 67(03):2008, 253–256.

3. Jemal, A, Siegel R, Xu J, et al. "Cancer Statistics 2010." *CA: A Cancer Journal for Clinicians.* 60 (5):2010, 277–300.

4. Adams, PE, Martinez, ME, Vickerie, JL, et al. "Summary Health Statistics for U.S. Adults: National Health Interview Survey, 2010." *Vital Health Statistics.* 251(10):2011, 1–117.

5. Jemal, A, Simard, EP, Dorell, C, et al. "Annual Report to the Nation on the Status of Cancer, 1975–2009, Featuring the Burden and Trends in Human Papillomavirus (HPV)-Associated Cancers and HPV Vaccination Coverage Levels." *Journal of the National Cancer Institute.* 105(3):2013, 175–201.

6. Howlader, N. Noone, AM, Krapcho, M, et al. (eds). "SEER Cancer Statistics Review, 1975–2010." Bethesda, MD: National Cancer Institute. www.seer.cancer. gov/csr/1975-2010 Retrieved 09/02/2013.

7. The American Cancer Society. "Cancer Facts & Figures 2014." www.cancer.org Retrieved 09/06/2014.

8. American Cancer Society Global Cancer Facts and Figures, 2nd Ed. Atlanta, GA: *American Cancer Society.* 2011.

9. Molina, JR, Yang, P, Cassivi, SD, et al. "Non-Small-Cell Lung Cancer: Epidemiology,

Risk Factors, Treatment, and Survivorship." *Mayo Clinic Proceedings.* 83(5):2008, 584–594.

10. Cornfield, J, Haenszel, W, Hammond, EC, et al." Smoking and lung cancer: recent evidence and a discussion of some questions." *International. Journal of Epidemiology.* 38(5):2009, 1175–1191.

11. Pope, CA, Burnett, RT, Thun, MJ, et al. "Lung Cancer, Cardiopulmonary Mortality, and Long-Term Exposure to Fine Particulate Air Pollution." *The Journal of the American Medical Association (JAMA).* 287(9):2002, 1132–1141.

12. Pope, CA, Dockery, DW. "Health Effects of Fine Particulate Air Pollution: Lines that Connect." *Journal of the Air & Waste Mangement Association.* 56:2006, 709–742.

13. U.S. Environmental Protection Agency. "Integrated Science Assessment for Particulate Matter." Environmental Protection Agency. 600/R-08/139F, 2009.

14. Darby, S, Hill, D, Auvinen, A, et. al. "Radon in homes and risk of lung cancer: collaborative analysis of individual data from 13 European case-control studies: Estimating lung cancer mortality from residential radon using data for low exposures of miners." *BMJ* (Formerly *British Medical Journal*). 330:2005, 223–233.

15. Howe, GR. "Lung Cancer Mortality between 1950 and 1987 after Exposure to Fractionated Moderate-Dose-Rate Ionizing Radiation in the Canadian Fluoroscopy Cohort Study and a Comparison with Lung Cancer Mortality in the Atomic Bomb Survivors Study." *Radiation Research.* 142(3):1995, 29–304.

16. Cardis, E, Gilbert, ES, Carpenter, L, et al. "Effects of Low Doses and Low Dose Rates of External Ionizing Radiation: Cancer Mortality among Nuclear Industry Workers in Three Countries." *Radiation Research.* 142(2):1995, 117–132.

17. Centers for Disease Control and Prevention & National Cancer Institute U.S. Cancer Statistics Working Group. Atlanta, GA, 2013. http://www.cdc.gov/uscs. Retrieved February 4, 2014.

18. McPherson, K, Steel, CM, Dixon, JM. " Breast cancer–epidemiology, risk factors, and genetics." *BMJ* (Formerly *British Medical Journal*). 321(7261):2000, 624–628.

19. Colditz, GA, Rosner, B. "Cumulative Risk of Breast Cancer to Age 70 Years According to Risk Factor Status: Data from the Nurses' Health Study." *American Journal of Epidemiology.* 152 (10): 2000, 950–964.

20. Marchbanks, PA, McDonald, JA, Wilson, HG, et al. "Oral Contraceptives and the risk of Breast Cancer." *The New England Journal of Medicine.* 346:2002, 2025–2032.

21. Rossouw, JE, Anderson, GL, Prentice, RL, et al. "Risks and benefits of estrogen plus progestin in healthy postmenopausal women: Principal results from the Women's Health Initiative randomized controlled trial." *The Journal of the American Medical Association (JAMA).* 288:2002, 321–333.

22. Hancock, SL, Tucker, MA, Hoppe, RT. "Breast Cancer After Treatment of Hodgkin's Disease." *Journal of the National Cancer Institute.* 85(1):1993, 25–31.

23. King, MC, Marks, JH, Mandell, JB, et al. "Breast and Ovarian Cancer Risks Due to Inherited Mutations in BRCA1 and BRCA2. *Science.* 302(5645):2003, 643–646.

24. Dumitrescu, RG, Cotarla, I. "Understanding breast cancer risk—where do we stand in 2005?" *Journal of Cellular and Molecular Medicine.* 9(1):2005, 208–221.

25. Key, J, Hodgson, S, Omar, RZ, et al. "Meta-analysis of Studies of Alcohol and Breast Cancer with Consideration of the Methodological issues." *Cancer Causes & Control.* 17(6):2006, 759–770.

26. Bianchini, F, Kaaks, R, Vainio, H. "Overweight, obesity, and cancer risk." *The Lancet Oncology.* 3(9):2002, 565–574.

27. American Cancer Society. Colorectal Cancer Facts & figures, 2011–2013. Atlanta, GA, American Cancer Society, 2011.

28. Siegel, R, Naidhadam, D, Jemal, A. "Cancer Statistics, 2012." *CA: A Cancer Journal for Clinicians.* 62(1):2012,10-29.

29. Edwards, BK, Ward, E, Kohler, BA, et al. "Annual report to the nation on the status of cancer, 1975-2006, featuring colorectal cancer trends and impact of interventions to reduce future rates." *Cancer.* 116(3):2010, 544–573.

30. Kirkegaard, H, Johnsen, NF, Christensen, J, et al. "Association of adherence to lifestyle recommendations and risk of colorectal cancer: a prospective Danish cohort study. *BMJ* (Formerly *British Medical Journal*). 341:2010, c5504.

31. Lynch, HT, de la Chapelle, A. "Hereditary colorectal cancer." *The New England Journal of Medicine.* 348(10):2003, 919–932.

32. Jasperson, KW, Tuohy, TM, Neklason, DW, et al. "Hereditary and familial colon cancer." *Gastroenterology.* 138(6):2010, 2044–2058.

33. Butterworth, AS, Higgins, J, Pharoah, P. "Relative and absolute risk of colorectal cancer for individuals with a family history: a meta-analysis." *European Journal of Cancer.* 42(2):2006, 216–227.

34. Bernstein, CN, Blanchard, JF, Kliewer, E, et al. "Cancer risk in patients with inflammatory bowel disease: a population-based study." *Cancer.* 91(4):2001, 854–862.

35. Larsson, SC, Orsini, N, Wolk, A. "Diabetes mellitus and risk of colorectal cancer: a meta-analysis. *Journal of the National Cancer Institute.* 97(22):2005, 1679–1687.

36. Huxley, RR, Ansary-Moghaddam, A, Clifton, P, et al. "The impact of dietary and lifestyle risk factors on risk of colorectal cancer: a quantitative overview of the epidemiological evidence." *International Journal of Cancer.* 125(1):2009, 171–180.

37. Cross, AJ, Ferrucci, LM, Risch, A, et al. "A large prospective study of meat consumption and colorectal cancer risk: an investigation of potential mechanisms underlying this association." *Cancer Research.* 70(6):2010, 2406–2414.

38. Neugut, AI, Jacobson, JS, Devivo, I. "Epidemiology of colorectal adenomatous polyps." *Cancer Epidemiology, Biomarkers & Prevention.* 2(2):1993, 159–176.

39. McCullough, ML, Robertson, AS, Chao, A, et al. "A prospective study of

whole grains, fruits, vegetables and colon cancer risk. *Cancer Causes and Control.* 14(10):2003, 959–970.

40. Cho, E, Smith-Warner, SA, Spiegelman, D, et al. "Dairy foods, calcium, and colorectal cancer: a pooled analysis of 10 cohort studies." *Journal of the National Cancer Institute.* 96(13):2004, 1015–1022.

41. Liang, PS, Chen, TY, Giovannucci, E. "Cigarette smoking and colorectal cancer incidence and mortality: systematic review and meta-analysis." *International Journal of Cancer.* 124(10):2009, 2406-2415.

42. Paskett, ED, Reeves, KW, Rohan, TE, et al. "Association between cigarette smoking and colorectal cancer in the Women's Health Initiative." *Journal of the National Cancer Institute.* 99(22):2007, 1729–1735.

43. Ferrari, P, Jenab, M, Norat, T, et al. "Lifetime and baseline alcohol intake and risk of colon and rectal cancers in the European prospective investigation into cancer and nutrition (EPIC)." *International Journal of Cancer.* 121(9):2007, 2065–2072.

44. Rothwell, PM, Wilson, M, Elwin, CE, et al. "Long-term effect of aspirin on colorectal cancer incidence and mortality: 20-year follow-up of five randomized trials." *The Lancet* 377(9759):2011, 3–4.

45. Hildebrand, JS, Jacobs, EJ, Campbell, PT, et al. "Colorectal cancer incidence and postmenopausal hormone use by type, recency, and duration in cancer prevention study II." *Cancer Epidemiology, Biomarkers & Prevention.* 18(11): 2009, 2835–2841.

46. Levin, B, Lieberman, DA, McFarland, B, et al. "Screening and surveillance for the early detection of colorectal cancer and adenomatous Polyps, 2008: a joint guideline from the American Cancer Society, the US Multi-Society Task Force on Colorectal Cancer, and the American College of Radiology." *CA: A Cancer Journal for Clinicians.* 58(3):2008, 130–160.

Chapter 7

1. Wang, Y, Beydoun, MA. "The Obesity Epidemic in the United States–Gender, Age, Socioeconomic, Racial/Ethnic, and Geographic Characteristics: A Systematic Review and Meta-Regression Analysis." *Epidemiologic Reviews.* 29 (1):2007, 6–28.

2. Wang, Y, Wang, JQ. "A comparison of international references for the assessment of child and adolescent overweight and obesity in different populations." *European Journal of Clinical Nutrition.* 56: 2002, 973–982.

3. U.S. Department of Health and Human Services, Public Health Service. *The Surgeon General's call to action to prevent and decrease overweight and obesity.* Rockville, MD: Office of the Surgeon General, 2001.

4. Centers for Disease Control and Prevention. "Prevalence of Obesity Among Adults: United States, 2011–2014." *NCHS (National Center for Health Statistics) Data Brief.* 131:2013. Data Brief 219(11): 2015, 1–4.

5. Ahima, RS, Lazar, MA. "The Health Risk of Obesity-Better Metrics Imperative." *Science.* 341:2013, 856–858.

6. de Gonzalez, B, Hartge, P, James, R, et al. "Body-Mass Index and Mortality among White Adults." *The New England Journal of Medicine.*364: 2011, 781–783.

7. Livingston, EH, Zylke, JW. "Progress in Obesity Research: Reasons for Optimism." *The Journal of the American Medical Association (JAMA).* 308(11): 2012, 1162–1164.

8. Flegal, KM, Carroll, MD, Kit, BK, et al. "Prevalence of obesity and trends in the distribution of body mass index among U.S. adults 1999–2010." *The Journal of the American Medical Association (JAMA).* 307(5) 2012, 491–497.

9. McTigue, KM, Garrett, JM, Popkin, MB. "The Natural History of the Development of Obesity in a Cohort of Young U.S. Adults between 1981 and 1998." *Annals of Internal Medicine.* 136:2002, 857–864.

10. Singh, GK, Kogan, MD, van Dyck, PC, et al. "A Multilevel Analysis of State and Regional Disparities in Childhood and Adolescent Obesity in the United States." *Journal of Community Health.* 33(2):2008, 90–102.

11. Lutfiyya, MN, Garcia, R, Dankwa, CM, et al. "Overweight and Obese Prevalence Rates in African American and Hispanic Children: An analysis of Data from the 2003–2004 National Survey of children's Health." *Journal of the American Board of Family Medicine.* 21(3):2008, 191–199.

12. Arner, P. "Obesity–a genetic disease of adipose tissue?" *British Journal of Nutrition.* 83(S1):2000, S9–S16. [Ed. Please verify exact name of this journal published by The Nutrition Society.]

13. Kim, B. "Thyroid Hormone as a Determinant of Energy Expenditure and the Basal Metabolic Rate." *Thyroid.* 18(2):2008, 141–144.

14. Bray, GA. "The Underlying Basis for Obesity: Relationship to Cancer." *The Journal of Nutrition.* 132(11):2002, 3451S–3455S.

15. Hill, JO, Peters, JC. "Environmental Contributions to the Obesity Epidemic." *Science.* 280(5368): 1998, 1371–1374.

16. Young, LR, Nestle, M. "The Contribution of Expanding Portion Sizes to the US Obesity Epidemic." *American Journal of Public Health.* 92(2):2002, 246–249.

17. Piernas, C, Popkin, BM. "Food Portion Size Patterns and Trends among U.S. Children and the Relationship to Total Eating Occasion, 1977–2006." *The Journal of Nutrition.* 141(6):2011, 1159–1164.

18. Bray, GA, Nielsen, SJ, Popkin, BM. "Consumption of high-fructose corn syrup in beverages may play a role in the epidemic of obesity." *The American Journal of Clinical Nutrition.* 79(4):2004, 537–543.

19. Piernas, C, Popkin, BM. "Snacking Increased among U.S. Adults between 1977 and 2006." *The Journal of Nutrition.* 140(2):2010, 325–332.

20. Blair, SN, Church, TS. "The Fitness, Obesity, and Health Equation: Is Physical Activity the Common Denominator?" *The Journal of the American Medical Association (JAMA).* 292(10):2004, 1232–1234.

21. Frank, LD, Andresen, MA, Schmid, TL. "Obesity relationships with community

design, physical activity, and time spent in cars." *American Journal of Preventive Medicine.* 27(2):2004, 87–96.

22. Morris, JN, Heady, JA, Raffle, PAB. "Coronary heart disease and physical activity of work." *The Lancet.* 262(6795):1953, 1053–1057.

23. Bray, GA. "Pathophysiology of Obesity." *The American Journal of Clinical Nutrition.* 55:1992, 488S–494S.

24. Bouchard, C, Bray, GA, Hubbard, VS. "Basic and clinical aspects of regional fat distribution." *The American Journal of Clinical Nutrition.* 52:1990, 946–950.

25. Allison,BD, Fontaine, KR, Manson, JE, et al. "Annual Deaths Attributable to Obesity in the United States." *Journal of the American Medical Association* (JAMA), 282(16): 1999, 1530-1538.

Chapter 8

1. Pollan, M. *In Defense Of Food: An Eater's Manifesto.* New York, NY: Penguin Group Inc., 2008.

2. Valtin, H. "Drink at least eight glasses of water a day." Really? Is there scientific evidence for "8 x 8"? *American Journal of Physiology. Regulatory, Integrative and Comparative Physiology.* 283:2002, R993–R1004.

3. Trichoppoulou, A, Cosacou, T, Bamia, C, et al. "Adherence to a Mediterranean diet and survival in a Greek population." *The New England Journal of Medicine.* 348:2003, 2599–2608.

4. Kreuter, MW, Brennan, LK, Scharff, DP, et al. "Do nutrition label readers eat healthier diets? Behavioral correlates of adults' use of food labels." *American Journal of Preventive Medicine.* 13(4):1997, 277–283.

5. Brandt, K, Molgaard, JP. "Organic agriculture: does it enhance or reduce the nutritional value of plant foods?" *Journal of the Science of Food and Agriculture.* 81(9):2001, 924–933.

6. Lee, IM, Paffenbarger, S. "Associations of Light, Moderate, and Vigorous Intensity Physical Activity with Longevity: The Harvard Alumni Health Study." *American Journal of Epidemiology.* 151(3):2000, 293–299.

7. Manson, JAE, Greenland, P, LaCroix, AZ, et al. "Walking Compared with Vigorous Exercise for the Prevention of Cardiovascular Events in Women." *The New England Journal of Medicine.* 347:2002, 716–725.

8. Kushi, LH, Fee, RM, Aaron, R, et al. " Physical Activity and Mortality in Postmenopausal Women." *The Journal of the American Medical Association (JAMA).* 277(16):1997, 1287–1292.

9. Tudor-Locke, C, Hatano, Y, Pangrazi, RP, et al. "Revisiting How Many Steps Are Enough?" *Medicine & Science in Sports & Exercise.* 195(08):2008, S537–S543.

10. Centers for Disease Control and Prevention. 2014 Surgeon General's Report: The

Health Consequences of Smoking–50 Years of Progress. http://www.cdc.gov/tobacco. Retrieved 02/20/2014.

11. Centers for Disease Control and Prevention Office on Smoking and Health, and National Center for Chronic Disease Prevention and Health Promotion. www.cdc.gov/tobacco. Retrieved 02/20/2014.

12. Taylor, DH, Hasselblad, V, Henley, J, et al. "Benefits of Smoking Cessation for Longevity." *American Journal of Public Health.* 92(6):2002, 990–996.

13. Oster, G, Colditz, GA, Kelly, NL. "The economic costs of smoking and benefits of quitting for individual smokers. *Preventive Medicine.* 13(4):1984, 377–389.

14. Glanz, K, Rimer, BK, Viswanath, K. (Eds.) *Health Behavior and Health Education: Theory, Research, and Practice.* San Francisco, CA: Josse-Bass, 2008.

15. Norman, P, Conner, M, Bell, R. "The theory of planned behavior and smoking cessation." *Health Psychology.* 18(1):1999, 89–94.

16. Michael, CF, Stevens, SS, Douglas, EJ, et al. "The Effectiveness of the Nicotine Patch for Smoking Cessation: A Meta-analysis." *The Journal of the American Medical Association (JAMA).* 271(24):1994, 1940–1947.

17. Lyna, P, McBride, C, Samsa, G, et al. "Exploring the association between perceived risks of smoking and benefits to quitting: Who does not see the link?" *Addictive Behaviors.* 27(2):2002, 293–307.

18. McElduff, P, Dobson, A, Beaglehole, R, et al. "Rapid reduction in coronary risk for those who quit cigarette smoking." *Australian and New Zealand Journal of Public Health.* 22(7):1998, 787–791.

19. Conoly, GN, Win, DM, Hecht, S, et al. "The reemergence of smokeless tobacco." *The New England Journal of Medicine.* 314:1986, 1020–1027.

20. Keith, CH, Vander, WM, DeBon, M, et al. "Smokeless Tobacco." *Preventive Medicine.* 32(3):2001, 262–267.

21. Hart, CL, Smith, GD, Hole, DJ, et al. "Alcohol consumption and mortality from all causes, coronary heart disease, and stroke: results from a prospective cohort study of Scottish men with 21 years of follow-up." *BMJ* (Formerly: *British Medical Journal*). 318:1999, 1725–1736.

22. Rimm, EB, Williams, P, Fosher, K, et al. "Moderate alcohol intake and Lower Risk of coronary Heart disease: Meta-analysis of effects on lipids and hemostatic factors." *BMJ* (Formerly *British Medical Journal*). 319:1999, 1523–1528.

23. Hiestand, DM, Britz, P, Goldman, M, et al. "Prevalence of Symptoms and Risk of Sleep Apnea in the US Population: Results From the National Sleep Foundation 'Sleep in America 2005 Poll.' *Chest Journal.* 130(3):2006, 780–786.

24. Patel SR, Ayas NT, Mark R, et al. "A Prospective Study of Sleep Duration and Mortality Risk in Women." *SLEEP.* 27(3):2004, 440-444.

25. Kripke, DF, Garfinkel, L, Wingard, DL, et al. "Mortality associated with sleep duration and insomnia." *Archives of General Psychiatry.* 59:2002, 131–136.

26. Qureshi, AI, Giles, WH, Croft, JB, et al. "Habitual sleep patterns and risk for stroke and coronary heart disease: A 10 year follow-up from NHANES I." *Neurology.* 48(4):1997, 904–910.

27. Folkman, S, Lazarus, RS. "An Analysis of Coping in a middle-aged Community Sample." *Journal of Health and Social Behavior.* 21(9):1980, 219–239.

28. Dimsdale, JE. "Psychological Stress and Cardiovascular Disease." *Journal of the American College of Cardiology (JACC).* 51(13):2008, 1237–1246.29. [Ed. Is the #29 supposed to be here?]

29. Schulz, R, Beach, S. "Caregiving as a risk factor for mortality: the caregiver health effects study." *The Journal of the American Medical Association (JAMA).* 282:1999, 2215–2219.

30. Spence, D, Barnett, PA, Linden, W, et al. "Recommendations on stress management." *The Journal of the American Medical Association (JAMA).* 160(9):1999, S46–S50.

31. Leahy, A, Clayman, C, Mason, I, et al. "Computerized biofeedback games: a new method for teaching stress management and its use in irritable bowel syndrome." *Journal of the Royal College of Physicians of London.* 32(6):1998, 552–556.

32. Granath, J, Ingvarsson, S, von Thiele U, et al. "Stress Management: A Randomized Study of Cognitive Behavioural Therapy and Yoga." *Cognitive Behaviour Therapy,* 35(1):2006, 3–10.

33. Grossman, P, Niemann, L, Schmidt, S, et al. "Mindfulness-based stress reduction and health benefits." *Journal of Psychosomatic Research.* 57(1):2004, 35–43.

34. Greeson, JM. "Mindfulness research update: 2008." *Journal of Evidence-Based Complementary and Alternative Medicine.* 14(1):2009, 10–18.

35. Link, BG, Phelan, J. "Social Conditions as fundamental Causes of disease." *Journal of Health and Social Behavior.* 51(1):2010, S28–S40.

36. Johnson, N, Backlund, E, Sorlie, PD, et al. "Marital Status and Mortality." *Annals of Epidemiology.* 10(4):2000, 224–238.

37. Seeman, TE. " Social ties and health: The benefits of social integration." *Annals of Epidemiology.* 1996, 442–451.

Chapter 9

1. Campos-Outcalt, D."The latest recommendations from the USPSTF." *The Journal of Family Practice.* 61(5):2012, 278–282.

2. Campos-Outcalt, D."The new cardiovascular disease prevention guidelines: What you need to know." *The Journal of Family Practice.* 63(2):2014, 89–93.

3. Wender, R,. Fontham, ET, Barrera, E, et al. "American Cancer Society Lung Cancer Screening Guidelines." *CA: A Cancer Journal for Clinicians*. 63(2):2013, 106–117.

4. Friedewald, SM, Rafferty, EA, Rose, SL, et al. "Breast Cancer Screening Using Tomosynthesis in Combination With Digital Mammography." *Journal of the American Medical Association (JAMA)*. 311(24):2014, 2499–2507.

5. Griffin, J. "Breast Cancer Screening." *Obstetric and Gynecological Practice Bulletin*. 122:2011, 1–11.

6. Saslow, D, Boetes, C, Wylie-Burke, C, et al. "American Cancer Society Guidelines for Breast Screening with MRI as an Adjunct to Mammography." *CA: A Cancer Journal for Clinicians*. 57:2007, 75–89.

7. Bernard, L, Lieberman, DA, McFarland, B. "Screening and Surveillance for the Early Detection of Colorectal Cancer and Adenomatous Polyps, 2008:? A Joint Guideline from the American Cancer Society, the US Multi-Society Task Force on Colorectal Cancer, and the American College of Radiology." *CA: A Cancer Journal for Clinicians*. 58:2008, 130–160.

8. Atkin, WS, Edwards, R, Kralj-Hans, I, et al. "Once-only flexible sigmoidoscopy screening in prevention of colorectal cancer: a multicenter randomized controlled trial." *The Lancet* 375 (9726):2010, 1624–1633.

9. Beydoun, HA, Beydoun, MA. "Predictors of colorectal cancer screening behaviors among average-risk older adults in the United States." *Cancer Causes & Control*. 19(4):2008, 339–359.

10. McTigue, KM, Harris, R, Hemphill, B, et al. "Screening and Interventions for Obesity in Adults: Summary of the Evidence for the U.S. Preventive Services Task Force." *Annals of Internal Medicine*. 139(11):2003, 933–949.

11. Ryan, DH, Braverman-Panza, J. "Obesity in Women," *The Journal of Family Practice*. 63(2):2014, S15–S20.

12. McTigue, KM, Garrett, J, Popkin, B. "The natural history of the development of obesity in a cohort of young U.S. adults between 1981 and 1998." *Annals of Internal Medicine*. 136:2002, 857–864.

13. Sturm, R, Hattori, A. "Morbid obesity rates continue to rise rapidly in the United States." *International Journal of Obesity*. 37(6):2013, 889–891.

14. Krebs, NF, Himes, JH, Jacobson, D, et al. "Assessment of Child and Adolescent Overweight and Obesity." *Pediatrics*. 120(S4):2007, 193–238.

Chapter 10

1. Seaquist, ER. "Addressing the Burden of Diabetes." *The Journal of the American Medical Association (JAMA)*. 311(22):2014, 226–2268.

2. Ross, Devol, Center for Health Economics at the Milken Institute. "An Unhealthy America: The Economic Burden of Chronic Disease." Presentation for Stakeholder

Forum, Santa Monica, CA: October 11, 2007. www.milkeninstitute.org Retrieved 04/08/2014.

3. Joyce, GF, Keeler, EB, Shang, B, et al. "The Lifetime Burden Of Chronic Disease Among The Elderly." *Health Affairs.* September 17:2005, 18—29. www. content. healthaffairs.org Retrieved 07/05/2014.

4. Lloyd-Jones, DM, Dyer, AR, Wang, R, et al. "Risk Factor Burden in Middle Age and Lifetime Risks for Cardiovascular and Non-Cardiovascular Death. " *American Journal of Cardiology.* 99:2007, 53–540.

5. CDC, NCHS. Underlying Cause of Death 1999-2013 on CDC WONDER Online Database, released 2015. Data are from the Multiple Cause of Death Files, 1999-2013, as compiled from data provided by the 57 vital statistics jurisdictions through the Vital Statistics Cooperative Program. Accessed Feb. 3, 2015. Retrieved from cdc. gov on May 25, 2016.

6. Stampler, J, Stampler, R, Neaton, JD, et al. "Low risk factor profile and long-term cardiovascular and non-cardiovascular mortality and life expectancy: findings for 5 large cohorts of young adult and middle-aged men and women." *The Journal of the American Medical Association (JAMA).* 282:1999, 2012–2018.

7. The National Cholesterol Education Program (NCEP). "Expert Panel on Detection, Evaluation, and Treatment of High Blood Cholesterol in Adults. Executive Summary of the Third Report." *The Journal of the American Medical Association (JAMA).* 285:2001, 2486–2497.

8. Fryar CD, Chen T, Li X. "Prevalence of Uncontrolled Risk Factors for Cardiovascular Disease: United States." 1999–2010[. NCHS data brief, no 103. Hyattsville, MD: National Center for Health Statistics. 2012.

9. Weiss, CO, Boyd, CM, Yu, Q, et al. "Patterns of prevalent major chronic disease among older adults in the United States." *The Journal of the American Medical Association (JAMA).* 298(10):2007, 1160–1162.

10. Rebecca L. Siegel, RL, Miller KD, et al. "Cancer Statistic2015."

CA: A Cancer Journal for Clinicians. 65(5): 2015, 29

11. Tinetti, ME, Fried, TR, Boyd, CM, et al. "Designing Healthcare for the Most Common Chronic Condition—Multi-morbidity." *The Journal of the American Medical Association (JAMA).* 307(23):2012, 2493–2494.

12. Wolff, JL, Starfield, B, Anderson, G. "Prevalence, expenditures, and complications of multiple chronic conditions in the elderly." Archives of Internal Medicine (italicize) 162 (20):2002, 2269-2276.

Summary

1. Stiefel MC, Perla RJ, Zell BL. "A Healthy Bottom Line: Healthy Life Expectancy as an Outcome Measure for Health Improvement Efforts." Milbank Quarterly. 88(1): 2010, 30–53.

Credits to Contributing Illustrators

The photo illustrations in the book were purchased by the authors with permission to use them in the book with attribution of credit to the respective illustrator and the company providing them. Following is the list of illustrations with corresponding attribution.

Figure 1 Stages of Atherosclerosis © Can Stock Photo Inc. /alila

Figure 2 Anatomy of a Heart Attack © Can Stock Photo Inc. /alila

Figure 3 Type-2 Diabetes Mechanism © Can Stock Photo Inc. /alila

Figure 4 X-Ray of Lung Cancer in Woman © Can Stock Photo Inc. /wonderisland

Figure 5 Stages in Breast Cancer © Can Stock Photo Inc. /alila

Figure 6 Colon Polyp © Can Stock Photo Inc. /Eraxion

Figure 7 Stages in Colon Cancer © Can Stock Photo Inc. /alila

About the Authors

Swarna Moldanado was born in India, and emigrated to the U.S. in 1977. She earned her undergraduate degree in nursing from Osmania University, Hyderabad, India, and a Masters degree from the University of Delhi, New Delhi. She obtained a second Masters degree in public health from the University of North Carolina, Chapel Hill, North Carolina. Her Ph.D. in nursing science was received from the University of Illinois in Chicago, Illinois. She has taught nursing, research method and public health in undergraduate and graduate programs in nursing in California and Illinois. She attained tenure at San Francisco State University, San Francisco, California, where she is a professor Emeriti. She has published articles in peer reviewed journals, and her first book, *Legumes: The Superfoods That Should Be Regulars On Your Plate,* was published in 2014 by Basic Health Publications.

Alex Moldanado was born and raised in Chicago, Illinois, where he also attended the medical school at the University of Illinois, Chicago Medical Center. He completed his post-graduate training in Family Medicine at Rush Presbyterian Medical Center in Chicago, Illinois. Following that, he served as a medical officer for a period of four years in the United State Navy. He later joined a small group of family physicians in private practice in San Mateo, California where he continues to practice today. Upon leaving active service in the Navy, he continued as a reservist for the next 20 years. He was recalled to active service during the second gulf war in 2003, and provided medical support to the 1st Marine Division in Iraq. He retired from the U.S. Navy as a reservist in 2008. In addition to seeing patients in his private practice, he is a volunteer physician at a free medical clinic, run by a nonprofit organization called the Samaritan House in San Mateo, California, and as well currently serves on its Board of Directors as a member.

The two authors, who are married to one another, live in Redwood City, California.

Index

Printed in the USA
CPSIA information can be obtained
at www.ICGtesting.com
JSHW012024140824
68134JS00033B/2856

9 781683 367888